Pediatric Critical Care

Editors

JERITHEA TIDWELL
BRENNAN LEWIS

CRITICAL CARE NURSING CLINICS OF NORTH AMERICA

www.ccnursing.theclinics.com

Consulting Editor
JAN FOSTER

June 2017 • Volume 29 • Number 2

ELSEVIER

1600 John F. Kennedy Boulevard • Suite 1800 • Philadelphia, Pennsylvania, 19103-2899

http://www.theclinics.com

CRITICAL CARE NURSING CLINICS OF NORTH AMERICA Volume 29, Number 2
June 2017 ISSN 0899-5885, ISBN-13: 978-0-323-53003-3

Editor: Kerry Holland
Developmental Editor: Colleen Dietzler

Photocopying

Single photocopies of single articles may be made for personal use as allowed by national copyright laws. Permission of the Publisher and payment of a fee is required for all other photocopying, including multiple or systematic copying, copying for advertising or promotional purposes, resale, and all forms of document delivery. Special rates are available for educational institutions that wish to make photocopies for non-profit educational classroom use. For information on how to seek permission visit www.elsevier.com/permissions or call: (+44) 1865 843830 (UK)/(+1) 215 239 3804 (USA).

Derivative Works

Subscribers may reproduce tables of contents or prepare lists of articles including abstracts for internal circulation within their institutions. Permission of the Publisher is required for resale or distribution outside the institution. Permission of the Publisher is required for all other derivative works, including compilations and translations (please consult www.elsevier.com/permissions).

Electronic Storage or Usage

Permission of the Publisher is required to store or use electronically any material contained in this periodical, including any article or part of an article (please consult www.elsevier.com/permissions). Except as outlined above, no part of this publication may be reproduced, stored in a retrieval system or transmitted in any form or by any means, electronic, mechanical, photocopying, recording or otherwise, without prior written permission of the Publisher.

Notice

No responsibility is assumed by the Publisher for any injury and/or damage to persons or property as a matter of products liability, negligence or otherwise, or from any use or operation of any methods, products, instructions or ideas contained in the material herein. Because of rapid advances in the medical sciences, in particular, independent verification of diagnoses and drug dosages should be made.

Although all advertising material is expected to conform to ethical (medical) standards, inclusion in this publication does not constitute a guarantee or endorsement of the quality or value of such product or of the claims made of it by its manufacturer.

Critical Care Nursing Clinics of North America (ISSN 0899-5885) is published quarterly by Elsevier Inc., 360 Park Avenue South, New York, NY 10010-1710. Months of issue are March, June, September, and December. Business and Editorial Offices: 1600 John F. Kennedy Blvd., Suite 1800, Philadelphia, PA 19103-2899. Periodicals postage paid at New York, NY and additional mailing offices. Subscription prices are $155.00 per year for US individuals, $385.00 per year for US institutions, $100.00 per year for US students and residents, $200.00 per year for Canadian individuals, $483.00 per year for Canadian institutions, $230.00 per year for international individuals, $483.00 per year for international institutions and $115.00 per year for Canadian and international students/residents. To receive student/resident rate, orders must be accompanied by name of affiliated institution, data of term, and the *signature* of program/residency coordinator on institution letterhead. Orders will be billed at individual rate until proof of status is received. Foreign air speed delivery is included in all *Clinics* subscription prices. All prices are subject to change without notice. **POSTMASTER:** Send address changes to *Critical Care Nursing Clinics of North America*, Elsevier Health Sciences Division, Subscription Customer Service, 3251 Riverport Lane, Maryland Heights, MO 63043. **Customer Service: 1-800-654-2452 (US and Canada); 314-447-8871 (outside US and Canada). Fax: 314-447-8029. E-mail:** JournalsCustomerService-usa@elsevier.com **(for print support) and** JournalsOnlineSupport-usa@elsevier.com **(for online support).**

Reprints. For copies of 100 or more of articles in this publication, please contact the Commercial Reprints Department, Elsevier Inc., 360 Park Avenue South, New York, New York, 10010-1710; Tel.: 212-633-3874, Fax: 212-633-3820, and E-mail: reprints@elsevier.com.

Critical Care Nursing Clinics of North America is covered in *MEDLINE/PubMed (Index Medicus), International Nursing Index, Nursing Citation Index, Cumulative Index to Nursing and Allied Health Literature, and RNdex Top 100.*

Contributors

CONSULTING EDITOR

JAN FOSTER, PhD, APRN, CNS
Formerly, Associate Professor, College of Nursing, Texas Woman's University, Houston, Texas; President, Nursing Inquiry and Intervention, Inc, The Woodlands, Texas

EDITORS

JERITHEA TIDWELL, PhD, RN, PNP-BC, PCNS-BC
NICU Clinical Nurse Specialist, Children's Health, Children's Medical Center Dallas, Dallas, Texas

BRENNAN LEWIS, MSN, RN, CPNP-PC/AC, PCNS-BC
Director, Patient Education and Engagement, Children's Health, Children's Medical Center Dallas, Dallas, Texas

AUTHORS

BONNIE ADRIAN, PhD, RN
Research Nurse Scientist, Clinical Informatics, University of Colorado Health, Colorado, Aurora, Colorado

ROBERT L. BOGUE, BS
Chief Executive Officer, Thor Projects LLC, Carmel, Indiana

TERRI L. BOGUE, MSN, RN, PCNS-BC
Clinical Nurse Specialist/Chief Operating Officer, Thor Projects LLC, Carmel, Indiana

CINDY DARNELL BOWENS, MD, MSCS
Critical Care Division, Associate Professor, Pediatrics, Medical Director, PICU, Patient Safety Officer, Children's Health, Children's Medical Center Dallas, Dallas, Texas

SHELLEY BURCIE, BSN, RN
Clinical Team Leader, Critical Care Services, Children's Health, Children's Medical Center Dallas, Dallas, Texas

CATHERINE CAMPESE, RN, MSN, CPNP
Nurse Practitioner, Chronic Pain Service, Children's Hospital of Pittsburgh, University of Pittsburgh Medical Center, Pittsburgh, Pennsylvania

KELLI CROWLEY, PharmD, BCPS, BCPPS
Pharmacist, Pharmacy, Children's Hospital of Pittsburgh, University of Pittsburgh Medical Center, Pittsburgh, Pennsylvania

DAYNA DOWNING, MHA, MBA
Program Manager, Simulation Lab, Children's Health, Children's Medical Center Dallas, Dallas, Texas

MELISSA GARCIA, RN, MSN, ACCNS-P
Department of Nursing, Children's Hospital of Philadelphia, Philadelphia, Pennsylvania

MICHELLE BORZIK GORETH, MSN, RN-BC, CPNP-AC, CCRN-P, CTRN, CPEN, TCRN
Adjunct Clinical Instructor, Pediatric Primary/Acute Care Nurse Practitioner Specialty Track, University of Alabama at Birmingham School of Nursing, Birmingham, Alabama; Lead Nurse Practitioner, Division of Pediatric Surgery, Department of Surgery, University of Mississippi Medical Center, Jackson, Mississippi

CYNTHIA GREENWELL, BSN, RN, CCRC
Children's Health, Children's Medical Center Dallas, Dallas, Texas

KRISTEN HOOD, BSRC, RRT-NPS
Clinical Educator, Respiratory Care Services, Children's Health, Children's Medical Center Dallas, Dallas, Texas

MARION KOPULOS, MSN, RN-BC
Board Certified Nursing Professional Development Specialist, Emergency Department and Intensive Care Unit, Children's Health, Children's Medical Center, Plano, Texas; Clinical Educator, Emergency Department and Intensive Care Unit, Children's Health, Children's Medical Center Dallas, Dallas, Texas

ALLISON LANGSTON, BSN, RN
Patient Safety Specialist, Quality, Children's Health, Children's Medical Center Dallas, Dallas, Texas

RACHEL LAUER, RN, MSN, FNP-BC
Nurse Practitioner, Chronic Pain Service, Children's Hospital of Pittsburgh, University of Pittsburgh Medical Center, Pittsburgh, Pennsylvania

BRENNAN LEWIS, MSN, RN, CPNP-PC/AC, PCNS-BC
Director, Patient Education and Engagement, Children's Health, Children's Medical Center Dallas, Dallas, Texas

ANN LUCKSTEAD-GOSDIN, MS, RN, CNS, CPNP-PC
Clinical Nurse Specialist, Children's Health, Children's Medical Center Dallas, Dallas, Texas

KAY MARTIN, BSRC, RRT-NPS
Simulation Educator, Simulation Program, Children's Health, Children's Medical Center Dallas, Dallas, Texas

HEIDI McNEELY, MSN, RN, PCNS-BC
Clinical Nurse Specialist, Inpatient Medical Unit, Children's Hospital Colorado, Aurora, Colorado

LAURA J. MISKE, RN, MSN, CNS
Department of Nursing, Children's Hospital of Philadelphia, Philadelphia, Pennsylvania

LYNN MOHR, PhD, APN, PCNS-BC, CPN
Assistant Professor/Associate Chair, Women, Children, Family Nursing and Director, Pediatric & Neonatal CNS Programs, College of Nursing, Rush University, Chicago, Illinois

JENNIFER PACKARD, MBA, MT (ASCP), SBB
Supervisor, Transfusion and Tissue Service, Children's Health, Children's Medical Center Dallas, Dallas, Texas

TRACY ANN PASEK, RN, MSN, DNP, CCNS, CCRN, CIMI
Clinical Nurse Specialist, Pain, Pediatric Intensive Care Unit, Evidence-Based Practice and Research, Children's Hospital of Pittsburgh, University of Pittsburgh Medical Center, Pittsburgh, Pennsylvania

CHRISTINE M. RILEY, BS, MSN, APRN, CPNP-AC
Nurse Practitioner, Division of Cardiac Critical Care Medicine, Children's National Health System, Washington, DC

JUDITH J. STELLAR, RN, MSN, CRNP, PPCNP-BC, CWOCN
Department of Nursing, Children's Hospital of Philadelphia, Philadelphia, Pennsylvania

MOLLY STETZER, RN, BSN, CWOCN
Department of Nursing, Children's Hospital of Philadelphia, Philadelphia, Pennsylvania

JODI THRASHER, MSN, RN, CFNP
Clinical Practice Specialist, Inpatient Medical Unit, Children's Hospital Colorado, Aurora, Colorado

JEFFERSON TWEED, BS
Children's Health, Children's Medical Center Dallas, Dallas, Texas

LORI VINSON, MSN, RN
Children's Health, Children's Medical Center Dallas, Dallas, Texas

CHARLES YANG, MD
Physician, Director of Anesthesia Pediatric Pain Management, Children's Hospital of Pittsburgh, University of Pittsburgh Medical Center, Assistant Professor, University of Pittsburgh School of Medicine, Pittsburgh, Pennsylvania

VIRGINIA B. YOUNG, MSN, RN, PCNS-BC
Emergency Services, Children's Health, Dallas, Texas

Contents

Preface: Bundles, Guidelines, Protocols, and More: A Pediatric Medley   xiii

Jerithea Tidwell and Brennan Lewis

Reducing Fresh Tracheostomy Decannulations Following Implementation of
a Fresh Tracheostomy Guideline   131

Kristen Hood, Brennan Lewis, and Cindy Darnell Bowens

> Pediatric patients undergoing tracheostomy placement are often medi-
> cally fragile with multiple comorbidities. The complexity of these patients
> partnered with the risks of a newly placed tracheostomy necessitates a
> clear understanding of patient management and clinical competence. At
> our institution, a quality improvement initiative was formed with a focus
> on increasing the safety of these patients by developing a postoperative
> care guideline.

Caring for Kids: Bridging Gaps in Pediatric Emergency Care Through Community
Education and Outreach   143

Ann Luckstead-Gosdin, Lori Vinson, Cynthia Greenwell, and Jefferson Tweed

> The Pediatric Emergency Services Network (PESN) was developed to
> provide ongoing continuing education on pediatric guidelines and
> pediatric emergency care to rural and nonpediatric hospitals, physi-
> cians, nurses, and emergency personnel. A survey was developed
> and given to participants attending PESN educational events to deter-
> mine the perceived benefit and application to practice of the PESN
> outreach program. Overall, 91% of participants surveyed reported
> agreement that PESN educational events were beneficial to their clin-
> ical practice, provided them with new knowledge, and made them
> more knowledgeable about pediatric emergency care. Education and
> outreach programs can be beneficial to health care workers' educa-
> tional needs.

Pediatric Mild Traumatic Brain Injury and Population Health: An Introduction for
Nursing Care Providers   157

Michelle Borzik Goreth

> Despite increasing injury prevalence of traumatic brain injury (TBI) in
> children, most injuries in children are mild in severity. Even mild injuries
> can result in long-term or chronic effects not apparent until the child
> ages, resulting in increased economic burden and overall lifetime costs
> related to injury. Early recognition of TBI is essential for ongoing evalu-
> ation and management of acute symptoms and reduction of chronic
> health effects. Providing early interventions to manage acute and post-
> concussive symptoms and reducing health disparities in children with
> mild TBI can minimize adverse events that impact health-related quality
> of life for the injured child and their family and increase overall popula-
> tion health.

When Nursing Assertion Stops: A Qualitative Study to Examine the Cultural
Barriers Involved in Escalation of Care in a Pediatric Hospital   167

Jodi Thrasher, Heidi McNeely, and Bonnie Adrian

Pediatric codes outside the ICU are associated with increased morbidity
and mortality. This qualitative research highlights results from confidential
interviews with 10 pediatric nurses with experience of caring for children
who required rapid response, code response, or transfer to intensive
care. Detailed examination of nurses' experiences revealed local factors
that facilitate and inhibit timely transfer of critical patients. Nurses identified themes including the impact of nurse assertiveness, providers' lack
of understanding of nursing, team communication, and other hospital cultural barriers.

Case Study of High-Dose Ketamine for Treatment of Complex Regional Pain
Syndrome in the Pediatric Intensive Care Unit   177

Tracy Ann Pasek, Kelli Crowley, Catherine Campese, Rachel Lauer, and
Charles Yang

Complex regional pain syndrome (CRPS) is a life-altering and debilitating
chronic pain condition. The authors are presenting a case study of a female who received high-dose ketamine for the management of her
CRPS. The innovative treatment lies not only within the pharmacologic
management of her pain, but also in the fact that she was the first patient
to be admitted to our pediatric intensive care unit solely for pain control.
The primary component of the pharmacotherapy treatment strategy plan
was escalating-dose ketamine infusion via patient-controlled-analgesia
approved by the pharmacy and therapeutics committee guided therapy
for this patient. The expertise of advanced practice nurses blended exquisitely to ensure patient and family-centered care and the coordination of
care across the illness trajectory. The patient experienced positive
outcomes.

Airways and Injuries: Protecting Our Pediatric Patients from Respiratory
Device-Related Pressure Injuries   187

Laura J. Miske, Molly Stetzer, Melissa Garcia, and Judith J. Stellar

Pressure injury prevention is required in all health care environments. Respiratory technology includes invasive and noninvasive positive pressure
ventilation methods of support and life-saving equipment. Pressure injury
can occur from tracheostomy tubes and their securement devices, or use
of noninvasive positive pressure ventilation interfaces or the head gear.
Methods instituted to decrease hospital-acquired pressure injury related
to noninvasive positive pressure ventilation and tracheostomy securement
devices are discussed.

Effective Management of Pain and Anxiety for the Pediatric Patient in the
Emergency Department   205

Virginia B. Young

Inadequate treatment of pain for children in the emergency department is a
persistent problem. Health care professionals are bound by ethical principles to provide adequate pain management; in children, this may be

challenging owing to cognitive and developmental differences, lack of knowledge regarding best practices, and other barriers. Studies have concluded that immediate assessment, treatment, and reassessment of pain after an intervention are essential. Self-report and behavioral scales are available. Appropriate management includes pharmacologic and non-pharmacologic interventions. Specific diagnoses (eg, abdominal pain or traumatic injuries) have been well-studied and guidance is available to maximize efforts in managing the associated pain.

Unbundling the Bundles: Using Apparent and Systemic Cause Analysis to Prevent Health Care–Associated Infection in Pediatric Intensive Care Units   217

Terri L. Bogue and Robert L. Bogue

Today's health care environment emphasizes patient outcomes, although financial incentives and penalties have placed a high priority on elimination of health care–associated infections (HAIs). The use of standardized care bundles is evidence-based; however, implementation of these bundles has not proven effective in eliminating HAIs. Actively learning from HAI events through the use of apparent and systemic cause analysis identifies new barriers to success and opportunities for improvement in further reducing HAIs. The effective use of apparent and systemic cause analysis requires a standardized review and is followed with the implementation of appropriate steps to remove newly identified barriers.

Putting the Family Back in the Center: A Teach-Back Protocol to Improve Communication During Rounds in a Pediatric Intensive Care Unit   233

Terri L. Bogue and Lynn Mohr

Patient- and family–centered care is endorsed by leading health care organizations. To incorporate the family in interdisciplinary rounds in the pediatric intensive care unit, it is necessary to prepare the family to be an integral member of the child's health care team. When the family is part of the health care team, interdisciplinary rounds ensure that the family understands the process of interdisciplinary rounds and that it is an integral part of the discussion. An evidence-based protocol to provide understanding and support to families related to interdisciplinary rounds has significant impact on satisfaction, trust, and patient outcomes.

Continuous Capnography in Pediatric Intensive Care   251

Christine M. Riley

Capnography or end-tidal carbon dioxide ($Etco_2$) monitoring has a variety of uses in the pediatric intensive care setting. The ability to continuously measure exhaled carbon dioxide can provide vital information about airway, breathing, and circulation in critically ill pediatric patients. Capnography has diagnosis-specific applications for pediatric patients with congenital heart disease, reactive airway disease, neurologic emergencies, and metabolic derangement. This modality allows for noninvasive monitoring and has become the standard of care. This article reviews the basic principles and clinical applications of $Etco_2$ monitoring in the pediatric intensive care unit.

Massive Transfusion Protocol Simulation: An Innovative Approach to Team Training   **259**

Allison Langston, Dayna Downing, Jennifer Packard, Marion Kopulos, Shelley Burcie, Kay Martin, and Brennan Lewis

At a 72-bed pediatric facility, a multidisciplinary team approach was used to prepare for the expansion of services for patients requiring spinal fusion. This preparation included emergency response requiring massive transfusion, necessitating the need for a Massive Transfusion Protocol (MTP) process to be in place. Such instances are low volume/high risk, creating difficulty for staff to gain and maintain proficiency with the equipment and processes related to the MTP in a secure environment. The purpose of this article is to highlight the preparation and education put into place before receiving the first pediatric patient for spinal fusion.

CRITICAL CARE NURSING
CLINICS OF NORTH AMERICA

FORTHCOMING ISSUES

September 2017
Hematologic Issues in Critical Care
Patricia O'Malley, *Editor*

December 2017
Pain Management
Stephen D. Krau and Maria Overstreet,
Editors

March 2018
Gastrointestinal Issues and Complications
Debra Sullivan and Deborah
Weatherspoon, *Editors*

RECENT ISSUES

March 2017
Infection in the Intensive Care Unit
Todd M. Tartavoulle and
Jennifer Manning, *Editors*

December 2016
**Mechanical Ventilation in the Critically Ill
Patient: International Nursing Perspectives**
Sandra Goldsworthy, *Editor*

September 2016
Cardiac Arrhythmias
Mary G. Carey, *Editor*

THE CLINICS ARE AVAILABLE ONLINE!
Access your subscription at:
www.theclinics.com

Preface

Bundles, Guidelines, Protocols, and More: A Pediatric Medley

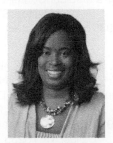

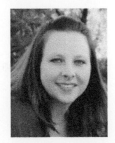

Jerithea Tidwell, PhD, RN, PNP-BC,
PCNS-BC

Brennan Lewis, MSN, RN, CPNP-PC/AC,
PCNS-BC

Editors

This special issue of *Critical Care Nursing Clinics of North America* is an assortment of relevant topics in pediatric critical care. The articles are written by experts from across the United States who are dedicated to bringing pediatric knowledge and innovation to the forefront. With the changes in the health care climate, clinicians must stay abreast of current evidence-based practices to ensure the highest quality of care. These articles are focused on keeping patients safe and improving patient outcomes through the use of standardized care approaches.

Bundles, guidelines, and protocols are common methods used to streamline health practices and are becoming increasingly more popular in pediatric care. These methods encourage clinicians to approach care using a systematic evidence-based process for medical decision making, therefore decreasing the risk of error in patient care and reducing the costs of unnecessary treatments. In this journal issue, you will find topics on the use of a guideline to reduce newly placed tracheostomy decannulations, the use of bundles to eliminate health care–associated infections, and how to effectively implement high-risk protocols.

Topics such as treatment of pain and anxiety in the pediatric intensive care and emergency department are addressed in this issue. The authors also discuss the vulnerability of the pediatric patient population and the importance of critical care across the continuum, and not just in a traditional intensive care or emergency room setting. During urgent situations, conscious thought may not be given to long-term patient effects following a traumatic injury. One of the articles in this issue takes a unique approach to pediatric trauma care by evaluating the need for clinicians to understand sequela following pediatric traumatic brain injury. Another article explains how to close the gaps in pediatric emergency care in nontraditional pediatric organizations through

Crit Care Nurs Clin N Am 29 (2017) xiii–xiv
http://dx.doi.org/10.1016/j.cnc.2017.04.001
0899-5885/17/© 2017 Published by Elsevier Inc.

ccnursing.theclinics.com

community education and outreach. Our hope is that reading the work of these authors will inspire others to develop similar practices and/or novelties in their practice organization.

Jerithea Tidwell, PhD, RN, PNP-BC, PCNS-BC
Children's Health
Children's Medical Center Dallas
Mailstop ST7.03
1935 Medical District Drive
Dallas, TX 75235, USA

Brennan Lewis, MSN, RN, CPNP-PC/AC, PCNS-BC
Children's Health
Children's Medical Center Dallas
Mailstop F2.19
1935 Medical District Drive
Dallas, TX 75235, USA

E-mail addresses:
Jerithea.Tidwell@childrens.com (J. Tidwell)
Brennan.Lewis@childrens.com (B. Lewis)

Reducing Fresh Tracheostomy Decannulations Following Implementation of a Fresh Tracheostomy Guideline

Kristen Hood, BSRC, RRT-NPS[a],*,
Brennan Lewis, MSN, RN, CPNP-PC/AC, PCNS-BC[b],
Cindy Darnell Bowens, MD, MSCS[c]

KEYWORDS

- Pediatric tracheostomy • Postoperative tracheostomy • Tracheostomy emergency
- Fresh tracheostomy • Tracheostomy guidelines

KEY POINTS

- Newly placed pediatric patients with tracheostomy are at high risk for morbidity in the immediate postoperative period.
- Managing an accidental decannulation in a patient with a newly placed tracheostomy requires a highly specialized skill set.
- Obtaining and maintaining competency in postoperative tracheostomy emergencies is a challenge.
- Standardized care guidelines, including emergency management for patients with a newly placed tracheostomy increases caregiver knowledge and patient safety.
- A quality improvement initiative at our institution led to the development of specific guidelines and an institutional reduction in newly placed tracheostomy decannulation.

The authors of this article do not have any commercial or financial conflicts of interest to report.
[a] Respiratory Care Services, Children's Health, Children's Medical Center Dallas, 1935 Medical District Drive, Dallas, TX 75235, USA; [b] Patient Education and Engagement, Children's Health, Children's Medical Center Dallas, 1935 Medical District Drive, Dallas, TX 75235, USA; [c] Critical Care Division, Pediatrics, PICU, Children's Health, Children's Medical Center Dallas, 1935 Medical District Drive, Dallas, TX 75235, USA
* Corresponding author.
E-mail address: Kristen.Hood@childrens.com

Crit Care Nurs Clin N Am 29 (2017) 131–141
http://dx.doi.org/10.1016/j.cnc.2017.01.001
0899-5885/17/© 2017 Elsevier Inc. All rights reserved.

ccnursing.theclinics.com

INTRODUCTION

Children undergoing tracheostomy placement are critically ill and have complex co-morbid conditions. The most common primary diagnoses on admission to critical care areas for these patients are related to respiratory, prematurity, neurologic, cardiovascular, oncologic, trauma, or vascular malformation conditions.[1] Additionally, the indications for tracheostomy placement are respiratory failure, aspiration, upper airway obstruction, and secretion management.[1–3] Given this high-risk population and their vulnerability, safety in the care of these children is imperative. For this reason, the immediate postoperative period following tracheostomy placement is spent in a critical care environment. This is because of the close monitoring and care required while the stoma is maturing into a healed tract, which takes approximately 5 to 7 days when placed in a controlled operative environment.[4] The term, fresh tracheostomy, or trach, is synonymous with newly placed tracheostomy. These terms are often used interchangeably when referring to patients who have just undergone the surgery for tracheostomy placement within the past 7 days.[4]

Nurses, respiratory therapists, intensive care providers, and surgeons must have a clear understanding and clinical competence of how to care for these patients in an emergency.[5] Emergencies with tracheostomies include accidental tube dislodgement or decannulation, tube obstruction, and hemorrhage.[3] Accidental decannulation in the fresh postoperative period is a significant emergency and a safety risk for the patient.[3] It is a challenge for health care providers to replace the trach due to the immature stoma tract, which differs from the procedure to replace a trach with a mature, well-formed stoma. It takes additional skill and expertise to safely care for this patient with this type of emergency. During the postoperative period, the surgical opening in the neck tissue has yet to fuse with the surgical opening in the trachea. If the tracheostomy tube is removed, the surgical opening in the trachea will close and reinsertion of the tube may require the use of sutures placed around the tracheal cartilage, called "stay sutures." These sutures when pulled are used to lift the trachea through the soft tissue and to align the opening in the trachea with the superficial incision. Tension placed on these sutures can reopen the trachea itself. The stay suture technique of tracheostomy is supported by the literature and is used at our institution.[6] Of note, a recent survey published by another pediatric hospital indicated that only 47% of nurses were completely comfortable changing a fresh trach.[5] Given that fresh trach emergencies are infrequent, it is also deemed to be a challenge to maintain the competence and comfort of any licensed health care provider in this situation.

One of the key measures to ensuring that emergencies do not happen is to have a well-defined care plan or guideline for this patient population. This includes having a sedation plan, proper securement of the tracheostomy, suction orders, and emergency equipment readily available at the patient's bedside, including spare trachs. Part of the care plan must include steps for managing fresh trach emergencies, should they occur. With these measures in place, trach emergencies can be prevented or managed effectively when they do occur, keeping the patient safe.

BACKGROUND

Children's Health, Children's Medical Center Dallas is a 487-bed, free-standing tertiary care pediatric hospital. In our institution, children with new tracheostomy tubes are cared for in the pediatric, neonatal, and cardiac critical care units until the first tracheostomy tube change has occurred. The standard of care is defined in a hospital policy related to the care and management of patients with tracheostomies. This policy includes the equipment required at the bedside for each tracheostomy patient and outlines the daily care practices for these patients. As a part of new employee orientation, nurses and respiratory therapists are taught indications for tracheostomy placement, postoperative management of fresh trachs, how to provide routine trach care, and emergency management. They also have a skills competency for the care of this patient population, although emergency trach management is simulated due to the limitation of using actual patients for training.

This institutional quality improvement initiative was preempted by 4 fresh trach decannulations in 2012 and 2013. Each of these events was entered into an electronic safety event reporting tool that is then reviewed by the institution's quality and safety department. In debriefing these events, several issues that challenged resolving the event were identified. This prompted a review of the hospital policies, guidelines, and protocols that addressed tracheostomy care, specifically care of the patient with a fresh tracheostomy. The review underscored the lack of clinical guidelines to direct the care of a patient with a newly placed tracheostomy.

METHODS

This quality improvement initiative did not require institutional review board approval or consent. A multidisciplinary team with representatives from Otolaryngology (ENT), Pediatric Surgery, Pediatric Critical Care, Neonatal Intensive Care, Respiratory Care, Nursing, and the Quality Department was developed. A charter was written describing the problem, objectives, scope, timeline, and deliverables of the project. The goal of this project was to cultivate guidelines for managing daily care of newly placed tracheostomy tubes and managing complications following newly placed tracheostomy tubes in pediatric patients. The aim for the project was to reduce the number of accidental decannulations in pediatric patients with newly placed tracheostomies. The current institutional care practices for patients following newly placed tracheostomies were ill defined in comparison with established tracheostomy care practices. A literature search was conducted to identify consensus on the care of fresh tracheostomies in pediatric patients. The following terms were used for the search: difficult airway, fresh trach care including adults, fresh trach emergencies, trach decannulation, and general tracheostomy care within the past 5 years. The search also included requests via list serves, personal and/or collegial contacts, and Internet searches. The search for literature and best practices revealed the following:

- Clinical Practice Guidelines
  - Children's Hospital of Orange County Fresh Tracheostomy Care Guideline[7]
  - The Royal Children's Hospital Melbourne Tracheostomy Management Guideline[8]
  - Tracheostomy Management Guideline[9]
- Expert Opinion/Consensus Statement
  - National Tracheostomy Safety Project[10]
  - Clinical Consensus Statement: Tracheostomy Care[1]
  - Accidental Decannulation Following Placement of a Tracheostomy Tube[11]

The team also reviewed peer institution policies related to care of tracheostomies in pediatric patients. The team completed a gap analysis between current practice and desired practice. Using the gap analysis, the team drafted clinical guidelines describing care for pediatric patients with newly placed tracheostomy. This guideline prescribed supplies to be kept at the bedside, daily assessment by the surgical and medical teams, and daily cares done by the bedside providers. In addition, the guideline provided detailed signage for posting at the bedside. The team also drafted an algorithm directing emergency care of the patient with a newly placed tracheostomy. After reaching consensus on the guidelines, order sets for the electronic medical record and videos for education of staff and caregivers were created.

FRESH TRACHEOSTOMY GUIDELINE COMPONENTS

The resulting guideline from the quality improvement initiative addresses the following key aspects of fresh tracheostomy care, which is defined as the care of the tracheostomy before the first tracheostomy change at which time the surgeon may deem the tract mature:

- Transition of care from the operating room (OR) to intensive care unit (ICU) team
- Daily ICU cares
- Emergency response

Goals for the protocol were as follows:

- Outline specific care of the patient with a fresh tracheostomy
- Develop care guidelines and restrictions to reduce accidental decannulation
- Provide expertise in emergency management through vetted evidence-based algorithms

BEDSIDE EQUIPMENT

Our institutional policy and procedure on the care of a patient with an established tracheostomy listed appropriate bedside equipment and supplies. Our consensus group identified additional items for the patient with a fresh tracheostomy. Key additions to bedside equipment included the following:

- Laceration tray intended for use in emergency removal of the tube in instances in which surgeons suture the trach tube flanges to the skin
- Fresh tracheostomy head-of-bed (HOB) sign (**Fig. 1**)

Our HOB sign for established tracheostomies lists the following:

- Tracheostomy size (inner diameter, outer diameter, and custom length, if applicable)
- Tracheostomy cuff status
- Suction catheter size and depth for suctioning
- Designated day of the week for trach tube change

Additions to the fresh tracheostomy HOB sign (see **Fig. 1**) were as follows:

- The name of the service that placed the tube was added to the fresh tracheostomy HOB sign to facilitate prompt notification in an emergency
- Two statements were added at the bottom of the sign, "I can be orally intubated with ET (endotracheal tube) size ___, and I can be bag-masked ventilated orally - Yes No."
- The last statement on the HOB sign is a reminder stating, "Two licensed personnel must be present for all patient manipulation, moves, and suctioning."

The American Academy of Otolaryngology recommends the contact of the placing service during a fresh tracheostomy emergency in their 2013 Clinical Consensus statement on tracheostomy care.[4] Both statements allow for bedside staff, including intensivists, to use the branching logic of the fresh tracheostomy emergency

Fresh Tracheostomy

My name is

_____

I have a

_____

(Tracheostomy size and brand)

_____

(cuff type and fill volume)

First Trach change by

_____

(Service that placed the tracheostomy)

Suction with

_____

(catheter size and depth for suctioning)

I can be orally intubated with ETT size ____
I can be bag masked ventilated orally   Yes   No

Two Licensed staff required for patient moves, manipulation, and suctioning

Fig. 1. Fresh tracheostomy HOB sign. (© 2016 Children's Health. All rights reserved.)

algorithms. The HOB location of this pertinent information saves precious time spent searching for ENT notes or awaiting surgical service answers. Attempting bag-mask ventilation for a patient without a patent upper airway provides no benefit while delaying proper therapy.[11] A patient in the initial postoperative period with significant airway pathology requires the timely reestablishment of artificial airway patency.[11] In such patients, short-term support through the upper airway via bag and mask will provide little assistance.[11]

When our quality initiative group reviewed the newly placed tracheostomy safety events, patient manipulation by a single licensed caregiver was identified as a potential root cause of events. Although key members of the patient's direct care team are likely aware of the patient's tracheostomy being newly placed; other critical care staff assisting at the bedside may benefit from a direct visual reminder. The presence of a warning statement regarding the need of 2 licensed staff for all patient manipulation in direct line of sight of caregivers will likely encourage staff to call for assistance before patient interventions. Although suctioning is the most frequent invasive procedure performed in ICUs, suctioning of a newly placed tracheostomy tube increases risk of dislodgement. At our institution, critical care staff has a high level of comfort in suctioning established tracheostomies, therefore readily identifying the increased risk of suctioning patients with fresh trachs was essential to increasing safety.

OPERATING ROOM TO INTENSIVE CARE UNIT TRANSITION

The OR to ICU transition is an essential opportunity to ensure a patient with a fresh tracheostomy is safe. Clear communication of the surgical procedure and findings, degree of difficulty of the trach placement, and sedation plans are important for hand-off and safe transfer of care. Our protocol addresses this transition under the section titled, "Immediate postoperative care to be completed by the Nurse or Respiratory Therapist."[12]

Key aspects of transition include the following:

- Ensuring stay sutures are present, labeled, and secured to the chest
- Assessment of security of tracheostomy ties
- Completion of the HOB sign
- Hanging of emergency algorithms
- Sedation discussion among the ICU and surgical team
- Patient restraint needs assessment

Key proactive tube patency measures that begin on ICU admission include the following:

- Immediate initiation of adequate humidification[4]
- Inline suction catheters used only for ventilated patients
  ○ Nonventilated patients use of inline catheters was prohibited to reduce the external pull or tension on the tube
- Presence of an order for suctioning frequency

If deficiencies are noted in handoff, they can be addressed in the moment versus waiting for surgical team response. The gathering of supplies, posting the HOB sign, and the corresponding emergency algorithms are all vital immediate cares. Prompt addition of optimal humidity is essential in reducing secretion viscosity. The loss of the normal upper airway function and its role in warming and humidifying inspired gas puts these patients at risk for mucous plugs following tracheostomy. The fresh surgical site increases serous and serosanguineous drainage in the trachea, increasing the need for suctioning immediately after trach placement. In addition to maintaining adequate humidity to optimize thinning of secretions, an ordered frequency for suctioning can assist in tube patency. At our institution, this frequency prompts the appropriate caregiver's presence at the bedside for the procedure and likely reduces the amount of unanticipated suctioning. Much of the initial work for the guideline is accomplished during this ICU admission process with a burden on the admitting providers to complete immediate cares and successfully begin the protocol.

DAILY CARES

Daily cares consisted of ensuring the immediate cares occurred and continued enhanced monitoring of the patient and tracheostomy. Nurses were designated to assess sedation level and tracheostomy tie security every 2 hours and as needed. In a recent prospective data analysis by White and colleagues,[11] mental changes including agitation were involved in 40% of accidental decannulations. Due to rapid changes in swelling, ties can quickly progress from tight to loose and vice versa. When tie security required manipulation of the ties, the service that placed the trach would be contacted.

In addition to monitoring of tie security, 2-hour assessments included evaluation of skin breakdown, bleeding, and crepitus of the neck and stoma area. Dressing changes and stoma care required the presence of 2 licensed providers. During suctioning, one provider holds the tube flanges stabilizing the airway while the second provider suctions. This is especially important during withdrawal of the catheter and the external pull on the tube must be offset. If resistance to catheter advancement was noted during suctioning, an ICU attending or fellow was notified. The most likely cause of resistance to suctioning is accumulation of dried secretions, serous fluid, and/or blood within the internal diameter of the tube.[3] Volume status, humidity, and suctioning frequency can be escalated to address resistance and may prevent the emergent change of a fresh tracheostomy tube due to plugging. The immediate loss of oral-nasal humidification from the upper airway, postoperative inflammation, and loss of effective cough function from bypassing of the larynx all contribute to risk of tube plugging in the patient with a fresh tracheostomy.[10] Moving of the patient was to occur after tie security was verified and a provider was designated to secure the flanges during the move.[4] Off-unit transports were evaluated for necessity and parents were not permitted to hold their children during this fresh postoperative stage.

EMERGENCY ALGORITHMS

Emergency algorithms were created to address the 2 most common tracheostomy events: accidental dislodgement (decannulation) and tube obstruction.[10] The suspicion of obstruction algorithm (**Fig. 2**) began with lavage and suction and then changing of an inner cannula if applicable.[4,9] Tracheostomies with inner cannulas allow for the changing of the internal lumen of the tube while the external portion of the tracheostomy tube remains in the trachea. These tracheostomies are only commercially available in large sizes and are referred to as dual cannula trachs. With dual cannula tubes, changing of the inner cannula will likely resolve obstruction while preserving the surgical site and maintaining airway stability. If the obstruction was still present after these initial interventions, staff called the service that placed the trach and the ICU attending. If the patient was stable, staff awaited instructions from the surgical service. If the patient was unstable, Anesthesia was consulted and staff proceeded to the dislodgement algorithm (**Fig. 3**). The dislodgment algorithm instructed staff to assess tube placement in the stoma by visualization and end-tidal carbon dioxide presence.[10] In the case of an unstable patient, if the patient could be bagged orally, the tube was removed after cuff deflation.[10] Then, while covering the stoma, oxygen and ventilation were provided via bag and mask.[10] These patients were designated as having a patent upper airway and traditional mask ventilation through the nasal oral route can achieve adequate support. If necessary, oral intubation was considered in these patients before surgical service intervention. Critical care and anesthesia providers are often experienced at establishing an airway through oral intubation; this could be considered in patients with patent upper airways in whom mask ventilation did not provide adequate support. For patients who could not be bagged from above and were unstable, the tube was removed and assistance provided with bag and mask to the stoma.[9,10] If this maneuver was ineffective at regaining patient stability, an attempt to replace the tube with the use of stay sutures was indicated. As with all emergent tracheostomy replacements, initially the same size was to be attempted followed by the next size down.[9] Ideally, the presence of the surgical service would occur before tracheostomy replacement. The surgical service will be most familiar with the method used to place the stay sutures as well as the proper procedure for using them to assist in opening and/or visualizing the surgical opening in the trachea.

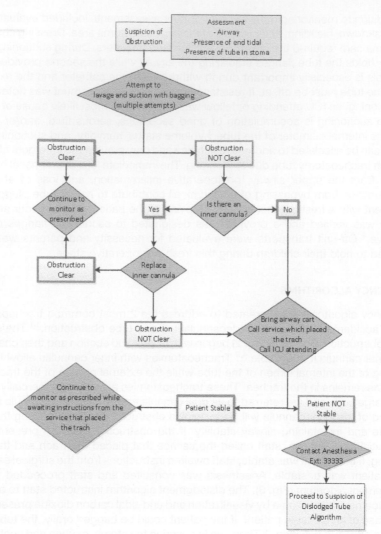

Fig. 2. Fresh tracheostomy emergency algorithm: suspicion of obstruction. (© 2016 Children's Health. All rights reserved.)

FRESH TRACH GUIDELINE IMPLEMENTATION

Our group recognized that an evidence-based multidisciplinary fresh trach guideline would experience little success without bedside staff awareness, competency, and compliance. True quality improvement is contingent on implementation as well as development. In 2015, Pritchett and colleagues[5] performed a cross-sectional analysis of survey data from inpatient nursing staff on comfort in managing acute and established tracheostomy tubes. The analysis focus was on identifying differences in nursing experience and primary unit work location as related to tracheostomy care comfort. Not surprisingly, the analysis revealed increased incidence of self-reported complete comfort in changing established tracheostomy tubes in nurses with 5 or more years of experience (60% vs 25% in nurse with <5 years' experience).[5] Although

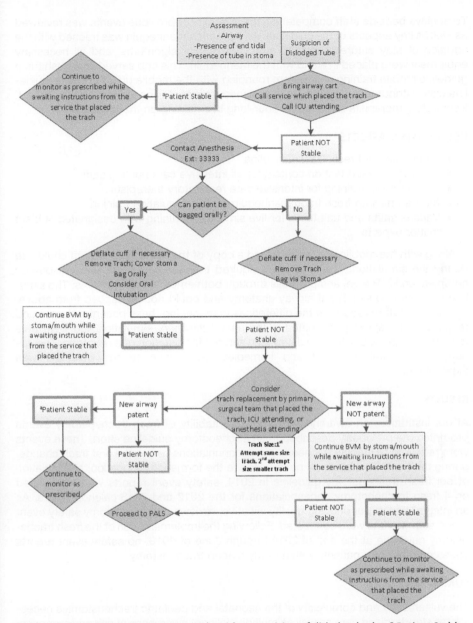

Fig. 3. Fresh tracheostomy emergency algorithm: suspicion of dislodged tube. [a] Patient Stable: Baseline hemodynamic status, Baseline oxygen saturation, Adequate ventilation, BVM, Bag valve mask; PALS, Pediatric Advanced Life support. (© 2016 Children's Health. All rights reserved.)

46% of the respondents overall were completely comfortable with established trach changes, a mere 4% of respondents were equally as comfortable managing an accidental decannulation in a fresh tracheostomy patient at C.S. Mott Children's Hospital.[5] Interestingly, Pritchett and colleagues[5] discovered no added comfort with accidental decannulation of a patient with a fresh tracheostomy with nursing years of experience.

To achieve bedside staff competency, the criticality of previous events was reviewed as well as key aspects of the guideline. An education mannequin was trached with the addition of stay sutures. An HOB sign, emergency algorithms, and all necessary equipment were placed in a crib with the mannequin. This crib served as a fresh trach guideline mobile training unit. Before rounding with the mobile unit, the official guideline was distributed and nursing staff assigned a computer-based test on the content. Respiratory therapists attended an hour-long live training on the guideline.

KEY TRAINING ASPECTS

- Distribution of Fresh Trach Guideline
- Computer-based test on content for all intensive care nursing staff
- One-hour live training for intensive care respiratory therapists
- Mobile unit with fresh trach mannequin for live simulation training
- Various shifts and unit times for live simulation training with designated subject matter experts

Along with the mobile unit, experts had a copy of the guideline that staff could use during the simulation. The simulation required the staff to list bedside equipment, complete an HOB sign, and progress through both emergency algorithms. The simulated patient had significant airway anatomy and could not be bagged from above, prompting staff to recognize the differences in managing these patients. Nurses and respiratory therapists participated in the multidisciplinary simulation and were able to witness experts pull the simulated stay sutures for insertion of a new tube. The education was well received and immediate adherence to the guideline was experienced.

RESULTS

At our institution, an awareness of the preventability of fresh tracheostomy events prompted the previously described fresh tracheostomy guideline effort. These events were reviewed to identify tracheostomy decannulations before the first trach change, during the fresh tracheostomy period. Before the formation, education, and initiation of our fresh tracheostomy guideline in 2014, safety event reports were completed on 4 fresh tracheostomy decannulations for the 2012 and 2013 calendar years. As an integral part of our ongoing quality initiative, reviews of tracheostomy safety event report submissions were conducted. Following the implementation of the fresh tracheostomy guideline at the end of 2014 through June of 2016, no safety event reports were completed for patients with a newly placed tracheostomy.

SUMMARY

The vulnerability and complexity of the neonatal and pediatric tracheostomies necessitates standardized care as well as multidisciplinary awareness of risk and response. The incidence of tracheostomy-related adverse events is difficult to track and international consensus groups have been active in the development of guidelines to prevent morbidity and mortality due to these events.[1] In the immediate postoperative period before the maturation of the tracheal stoma, adverse events yield a higher likelihood of morbidity and mortality.[12] These medically complex patients are particularly fragile during the postoperative tracheostomy period. The smaller size and length of pediatric tracheostomy tubes lends to easier accidental dislodgment and tube obstruction.

At our institution, the care of patients with a fresh trach was at best loosely outlined. The quality improvement initiative sought to improve institutional awareness and knowledge with the development of a fresh tracheostomy guideline. This guideline addressed key aspects of daily nursing and respiratory care as well as emergency response. A large multidisciplinary group developed, reviewed, and approved the guideline. Education was provided in a live interactive format that required the use of the emergency algorithms. These guidelines are available to our institution's staff at the bedside via an internal Web-based application. The HOB sign and emergency algorithms are available to print in the application; laminated copies are kept in the ICUs as well. This quality improvement initiative achieved our institutional goal of reduction in fresh tracheostomy decannulations. The continued monitoring of safety events is necessary as well as a plan for ongoing competency of bedside staff.

REFERENCES

1. Lavin J, Shah R, Greenlick H, et al. The global tracheostomy collaborative: one institute's experience with a new quality improvement initiative. Int J Pediatr Otorhinolaryngol 2016;80:106–8.
2. Lawrason A, Kavanagh K. Pediatric tracheotomy: are the indications changing? Int J Pediatr Otorhinolaryngol 2013;77:922–5.
3. Morris LL, Whitmer A, McIntosh E. Tracheostomy care and complications in the intensive care unit. Crit Care Nurse 2013;33(5):18–30.
4. Mitchell RB, Hussey HM, Setzen G, et al. Clinical consensus statement: tracheostomy care otolaryngology. Head Neck Surg 2013;148(1):6–20.
5. Pritchett CV, Rietz Foster M, Ray A, et al. Inpatient nursing and parental comfort in managing pediatric tracheostomy care and emergencies. JAMA Otolaryngol Head Neck Surg 2016;142(2):132–7.
6. Lee SH, Kim KH, Woo SH. The usefulness of stay suture technique in tracheostomy. Laryngoscope 2015;125:1356–9.
7. Children's Hospital of Orange County. Fresh tracheostomy care guideline. 2014. Available at: http://www.choc.org/wp/wpcontent/uploads/careguidelines/Fresh TracheostomyCareGuideline.pdf. Accessed August 30, 2016.
8. The Royal Children's Hospital Melbourne. Tracheostomy management. 2014. Available at: http://www.rch.org.au/rchcpg/hospital_clinical_guideline_index/ Tracheostomy_Management_Guidelines/. Accessed September 1, 2016.
9. McGrath BA, Bates L, Atkinson D, et al. Multidisciplinary guidelines for the management of tracheostomy and laryngectomy airway emergencies. Anaesthesia 2012;67:1025–41.
10. National Tracheostomy Safety Project. NTSP manual 2013. 2013. Available at: http://www.tracheostomy.org.uk/Resources/Printed%20Resources/NTSP_Manual_2013.pdf. Accessed September 1, 2016.
11. White AC, Purcell E, Urquhart MB, et al. Accidental decannulation following placement of a tracheostomy tube. Respir Care 2012;57(12):2019–25.
12. Children's Health, Children's Medical Center. Fresh tracheostomy clinical protocol. 2015. Available via internal Web-based application. Accessed August 30, 2016.

Caring for Kids

Bridging Gaps in Pediatric Emergency Care Through Community Education and Outreach

Ann Luckstead-Gosdin, MS, RN, CNS, CPNP-PC*, Lori Vinson, MSN, RN, Cynthia Greenwell, BSN, RN, CCRC, Jefferson Tweed, BS

KEYWORDS

- Outreach • Pediatric emergency care • Trauma • Education

KEY POINTS

- A dedicated Education and Outreach program was developed to improve emergency care of pediatric patients.
- A Quality Survey Assessment of the Education and Outreach program revealed more than 91% of participants agreed the program was beneficial and provided new knowledge.
- Providing specialty education has had a positive impact on establishing collaborative relationships and communication with local health care providers and will likely contribute to improved patient care and a reduction of cost.

INTRODUCTION

In 1913, the American College of Surgeons (ACS) was founded based on the desire to improve the care received by surgical patients and to provide education to surgeons.[1]

Then in 1922, Charles L. Scudder, MD, FACS, established the ACS Committee on Trauma (ACS-COT) whose purpose is to improve the care of injured patients.[1] They accomplish this by designating Trauma Systems of Care that provide optimal care by using the Trauma Systems' available resources.

Receiving care at a Pediatric Trauma Center (PTC) has been associated with lower mortality rates and improved outcomes for injured children.[2] However, up to 90% of injured children do not receive care at a PTC, and will receive care at a nonchildren's hospital due to limited resources and lack of pediatric surgeons and specialists in a given region. This lack of resources has led to the development of academic-community partnerships in Pediatric Trauma Care. Kelley-Quon and colleagues[2] concluded that these academic-community partnerships have been shown to be a

Children's Health^{SM} Children's Medical Center, Dallas, TX, USA
* Corresponding author. Children's Medical Center Plano, 7601 Preston Road, Office L1270, Plano, TX 75024.
E-mail address: ann.gosdin@childrens.com

Crit Care Nurs Clin N Am 29 (2017) 143–155
http://dx.doi.org/10.1016/j.cnc.2017.01.002
0899-5885/17/© 2017 Elsevier Inc. All rights reserved.

feasible alternative that may lead to improved outcomes.[2] Therefore, it is imperative that PTCs partner with the community, adult, and rural hospitals to provide education on optimal pediatric emergency and trauma care.[3,4]

The American Academy of Pediatrics Committee on Pediatric Emergency Medicine reports that young adults and children ages 24 years and younger have been shown to use emergency medical services (EMS) less often than adults, accounting for approximately 10% of prehospital emergency responses and 37% of emergency department visits.[5] Because there are a lower number of pediatric patients seen in the prehospital setting, nonpediatric facilities, and in rural settings, it is difficult for staff at nonpediatric facilities to maintain their skills related to pediatric care. This leads to an increased risk of the pediatric population not receiving the appropriate intervention, such as proper cervical spine immobilization and splinting, because the nonpediatric center might not have equipment solely made for children. Additional challenges include lack of access to higher levels of care for EMS for children, especially in rural areas. Therefore, adult centers frequently transfer pediatric patients to a local children's hospital due to lack of knowledge, and reported anxiety about care for the pediatric patient. When pediatric patients are seen at an adult center and then transferred to a pediatric facility, there is an increase in cost and the use of resources for the patient, the patient's family, and the health care system overall. Therefore, providing education and support to adult facilities is important so they are better able to manage less complex pediatric conditions and avoid having to transfer the infant or child to a specialty pediatric facility. This would help reduce costs and provide a more efficient use of resources.

According to Curran and colleagues,[6] rural physicians play a key role in the initial emergency management of trauma and report a higher need for continuing education on pediatric emergencies and procedures as compared with urban physicians. Because of the lack of resources, rural physicians report the need to perform a wide range of procedural skills, which requires them to maintain competency in a number of advanced clinical areas, such as emergency medicine and pediatrics. Rural physicians report they often do not feel sufficiently prepared to perform these advanced clinical skills and procedures and must work more independently than urban physicians without ready access to the latest medical technology and specialist consultation.[6-8]

As early as 1997, continuing education to rural nurses has also shown to be beneficial.[9,10] One trauma center at Denver Health Medical Center (DHMC) integrated rural nursing education into an existing medical outreach program that provided trauma education. The DHMC rural nursing outreach program combined both didactic and clinical instruction on critical care and trauma courses based on the nurses' identified educational needs. Evaluation by participants of the DHMC outreach program to rural nurses reported that the program improved communication, improved collaboration with other health care workers, and was beneficial to trauma patients across the continuum of care.[11]

Paulson[12] described another rural outreach program for emergency nurses called the Emergency Nurses Partnership Program (ENPP), which was developed by West Virginia University in an effort to address barriers to continuing education for their rural nurses. The West Virginia ENPP combined both didactic and clinical instruction on emergency care and trauma to rural communities. Participants of the ENPP reported that they believed that the combined didactic and interactive precepted sessions made a positive contribution to trauma and emergency care in that geographic area.[12]

The Pediatric Level I Trauma Center at Children's Medical Center Dallas, the flagship of Children's Health, established The Pediatric Emergency Services Network (PESN). PESN was created to serve as a resource to provide leadership in evidence-based pediatric emergency education, pediatric trauma education, and outreach to the community. PESN was selected and received a grant as a special multiyear Signature Project from The Crystal Charity Ball in 2005. PESN began as a network that included affiliates from 6 not-for-profit hospitals in the local Dallas, Texas, area, and the paramedic/emergency medical technician (EMT) student program at the University of Texas Southwestern Medical Center (UT Southwestern). Continuing education offerings were provided on a quarterly basis at no cost to participants and an all-day conference was offered on an annual basis for a minimal fee. Contracts were made between network hospitals to provide funding toward pediatric care for each of the affiliates. Topics for the educational events were chosen by the different hospitals within PESN and requested topics listed on continuing education evaluation summaries from participants at PESN educational events.

Requests for continuing education were also received by the community. Education requests were made by other local nonpediatric hospitals outside of PESN, rural hospitals, the Children's Medical Center School Nurse Committee, and other community organizations. Examples of the most requested outreach education topics by non-pediatric and rural facilities included child abuse, pediatric trauma, emergency care of pediatric patients, and family presence during resuscitation. Initially, the PESN coordinator served as the liaison for the PESN affiliates and helped facilitate the education requests for PESN affiliates and the community. In 2011, the PESN Clinical Nurse Specialist (CNS) was added to the PESN program to also serve as a liaison and help facilitate education and outreach requests for PESN.

In 2013, the PESN program grew and expanded the PESN coordinator role by having a paramedic serve as the liaison for EMS. This new role assisted with PESN education and outreach efforts and also included education of students at different paramedic schools in the local community. In 2016, the paramedic role was expanded further and changed to the PESN EMS program manager. The PESN EMS program manager facilitates education of paramedic students and reviews prehospital care of pediatric patients transferred into Children's Health. The PESN EMS program manager also serves as a liaison for EMS, and helps facilitate PESN outreach and education efforts.

In July of 2013 the PESN model changed and focused on traveling to rural communities to provide education instead of having quarterly education events in the Dallas-Fort Worth area. This revised program model led to a decrease in the number of large community educational events from 4 events a year to 2 events a year. The main focus of PESN is to provide information on evidence-based interventions for pediatric care and professional practice guidelines for pediatric emergency care. The PESN also assists hospitals with obtaining resources to develop their own policies and clinical practice guidelines for pediatric patients at their institution. Additionally, PESN provides assistance to the school nurse community with obtaining protocols and clinical practice guidelines for emergency care of pediatric patients in the school setting.

In an effort to determine the quality and effectiveness of the PESN outreach program, it was determined that the program should be evaluated by the participants and facilities that received outreach and education from PESN. It was important to determine the perceived benefit of the program and the perceived application to clinical practice. Validation of the benefits of the PESN program also could ensure the continued efforts for providing optimal pediatric care both locally and on a regional level.

METHODS

To determine the perceived benefit and application of the PESN outreach program, a survey was crafted with consultation of the Trauma Research Team at Children's

Medical Center Dallas. A literature search was performed to determine if there were any existing instruments that could be used and it was concluded that there were no tools available that would cover our specific topics. The survey and project summary were submitted to and evaluated by the UT Southwestern institutional review board (IRB) for review. The IRB determined this project did not meet the definition of human subject research and no IRB approval or oversight was required.

Survey assessments were conducted at PESN educational events from May 15, 2015, to May 31, 2016. Educational events were advertised and promoted by e-mail to individuals who attended previous PESN educational events or to individuals who asked to be on the PESN e-mail list for further educational offerings. Educational events also were advertised on the continuing education conference Web page of Children's Health. The marketing department also assisted with managing the e-mail list and promoting the event. A copy of the survey used can be seen in Appendix 1.

All participants were offered an electronic version or paper version of the survey at the beginning of each presentation. The announcement that included instructions and an explanation about the purpose of the survey was given to the participants of each PESN educational event. It was made clear that all participation was voluntary and there would be no compensation, but that the data from the surveys would contribute to the improvement of future educational events offered by PESN. As the surveys were anonymous, it was up to the attendee to indicate if they had previously turned in a survey for the event. If the attendee attended more than 1 event in the survey time frame, he or she was asked to fill out a survey at every event, as their views may have changed and there were questions pertaining to each specific event they attended.

The survey collected comments with simple "fill-in-the-circle" anonymous responses. The survey was designed to collect the participants' perceptions as well as their demographic information, including gender, ethnic/racial background, educational level, and length of time in current health care/educational career. Data were also collected on the type of certifications and or licenses held, and the number of PESN events attended to date. Participants were asked to rank their impressions of the educational events they attended by using a 5-point Likert scale ranking their agreement from strongly disagree to strongly agree (see Appendix 1). The current educational event was evaluated to determine if the education event provided new knowledge about pediatric emergency care and if the information provided at the event would be used in the participants' clinical practice. The overall impression of the PESN program was evaluated by asking participants if the educational events benefited their clinical practice, increased their knowledge about pediatric emergency care, and if they would recommend PESN education events to their colleagues.

All submissions were collected into the UT Southwestern Research electronic data capture (REDCap) system. The Trauma Research Team chose the REDCap system for data collection because of its robust data capturing and security capabilities. REDCap is a novel software program designed for rapid development and deployment of electronic data capture tools to support clinical and translational research.[13] UT Southwestern has a REDCap implementation that is supported by a National Institutes of Health (NIH) grant (Clinical and Translational Science Award NIH Grant UL1TR001105). Through existing research collaboration between UT Southwestern and Children's Health, PESN was able to use the survey feature for this study. Results were reviewed by the PESN team, including the senior director over PESN, Trauma, and EMS. Results were also shared with the Trauma Medical Director, and the PESN and Trauma Services Department Performance Improvement teams.

Sample

The population surveyed included a convenience sample of teaching professionals, health care providers, emergency personnel, and health care students who attended PESN educational events. Electronic surveys were offered for the first 3 events, but were not offered at later events because of the low response rate in electronic form. All paper copies were entered manually into the REDCap database and a random sample was reviewed to ensure accuracy. Only 1 team member had administrative access to the REDCap system for survey administration. All survey responses were kept anonymous and were represented by a nonidentifying number within the REDCap system.

To maintain confidentiality during analysis and presentation, subgroups of each demographic captured in the survey were combined to ensure each group consisted of at least 10 members. Provider subgroups consisted of prehospital providers (EMT, Emergency Medical Technician-Intermediate [EMT-I], Emergency Medical Technician-Paramedic [EMT-P]), nurses (licensed vocational nurse, registered nurses [RN]), practitioner (physicians and advanced practice providers, which includes advanced practice nurses and physician assistants), and other (respiratory therapist or no certification listed). Race subgroups consisted of Asian, Black, White, and other (American Indian, Alaskan Native, mixed race, or no response). Education level was classified by the highest education achieved, including no college degree (high school or some college), associate's degree, bachelor's degree, and graduate degree or higher (graduate degree or doctorate). The number of previously attended events was classified as no previous events, 1 to 3 events, 4 to 6 events, or 7 or more events.

To maintain adequate sample sizes for comparison based on response demographics, the Likert scale responses were divided into 2 categories: positive agreement (Agree, Strongly Agree) or no agreement (No Response, Neutral, Disagree, Strongly Disagree). Descriptive statistics were used to describe the sample population. Counts and proportions were used to describe the data captured on the survey form. Chi-square and Fisher exact tests where appropriate were used to compare correlation between nonordinal count variables. Python version 2.7.10 (Beaverton, OR) running on Enthought Canopy version 1.6.2 (Austin, TX) was used for data preparation and analysis.

Results

During the study time frame there were total of 6 different educational offerings. A total of 240 participants signed in during registration. The total number of surveys returned was 169 (70.4%) from all 6 events. The response rate for the first 3 event surveys administered on paper was significantly higher than for surveys administered online (73.6% vs 52.5%, $P = .01$). No difference exists in the types of providers that registered for events in comparison with the returned surveys (**Fig. 1**). Most respondents were RNs who had more than 10 years of health care experience. The demographics of the respondents can be seen in **Table 1**. Ethnicity was left blank for 3% (n = 5) of the survey responses, and race was left blank for approximately 2% (n = 3) of the survey responses. The rest of the demographic data responses were complete for each survey received.

Overall responses to questions evaluating the PESN with regard to the current event attended, and the PESN as a whole are displayed in **Table 2**. Evaluation of the PESN educational event most currently attended showed that most (91.1%) of the responses were positive (62.1% strongly agreed and 29.0% agreed) that PESN provided educational offerings and imparted new knowledge about pediatric emergency care.

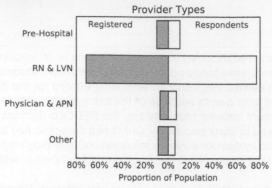

Fig. 1. Types of providers that registered for events versus the returned surveys. APN, Advanced Practice Nurse.

Table 1 Respondent demographics	
	n (%)
n	169
Women (%)	138 (81.7)
Ethnicity	
Hispanic or Latino	16 (9.5)
Not Hispanic or Latino	148 (87.6)
Race	
Asian	12 (7.1)
Black	13 (7.7)
White	131 (77.5)
Other	10 (5.9)
Health care experience	
New to role	11 (6.5)
1–3 y	18 (10.7)
4–6 y	26 (15.4)
7–10 y	26 (15.4)
>10 y	87 (51.5)
Highest education	
No degree	12 (7.1)
Associate's degree	27 (16.0)
Bachelor's degree	103 (60.9)
Graduate degree or higher	27 (16.0)
Certifications	
Prehospital	17 (10.1)
Registered nurse	130 (76.9)
Physician and advanced practice provider	12 (7.1)
Other	10 (5.9)
Number of past events attended	
None	83 (49.1)
1–3 events	47 (27.8)
4–6 events	21 (12.4)
>7 events	17 (10.1)

Table 2 Evaluation of current event and PESN as a whole						
	NR n (%)	SD n (%)	D n (%)	N n (%)	A n (%)	SA n (%)
Current PESN Event						
Educational event provided new knowledge about pediatric emergency care	9 (5.3)	1 (0.6)	0 (0.0)	5 (3.0)	49 (29.0)	105 (62.1)
Plan to use the information learned at this educational event in clinical practice	10 (5.9)	1 (0.6)	0 (0.0)	5 (3.0)	54 (32.0)	99 (58.6)
PESN as a whole						
The education that PESN provides benefits clinical practice	10 (5.9)	1 (0.6)	1 (0.6)	3 (1.8)	59 (34.9)	95 (56.2)
More knowledgeable about pediatric emergency care because of PESN	10 (5.9)	1 (0.6)	0 (0.0)	4 (2.4)	58 (34.3)	96 (56.8)
Would recommend PESN events to colleagues	9 (5.3)	1 (0.6)	0 (0.0)	5 (3.0)	48 (28.4)	106 (62.7)

Abbreviations: A, agree; D, disagree; N, neutral; NR, no response; PESN, Pediatric Emergency Services Network; SA, strongly agree; SD, strongly disagree.

Most (90.6%) respondents also positively agreed (58.6% strongly agreed and 32.0% agreed) that they would use the new information they learned at the specific PESN educational event in their clinical practice.

When responding about the PESN program overall, most (91.1%) respondents positively agreed (56.2% strongly agreed and 34.9% agreed) the education provided by PESN benefited their clinical practice. Most (91.1%) respondents also positively agreed (56.8% strongly agree, 34.3% agree) they felt more knowledgeable about providing pediatric emergency care because of education provided by PESN. Overall, 91.1% of participants positively agreed (62.7% strongly agree, 28.4% agree) they would recommend PESN events to their colleagues.

Fewer than 6% (n = 10) did not provide a response in any of the evaluation categories. In an effort to achieve conservative estimates, the nonresponses were maintained in the denominator population when calculating proportions of positive responses.

The proportions of positive responses for each survey domain stratified by each of the demographic classifications of the study population are displayed in **Fig. 2**. Columns separate the question domains from the survey, and rows separate the different demographic strata in the dataset. Darker color indicates a lower proportion of positive responses and lighter color indicates more positive responses within each survey domain for each demographic stratum. Data are presented as percentage of responses that were positive within each stratum.

There is no discernible pattern in the years of experience and the evaluation of the PESN, with most responses being positive across all domain questions (see **Fig. 2**A). Persons with no college degree tended to evaluate PESN lower across all domains (see **Fig. 2**B). A Fisher exact test shows a trend toward fewer positive survey responses from this subgroup with regard to PESN providing new knowledge (75% positive, $P = .286$), and use of information in clinical practice (67% positive, $P = .061$). A

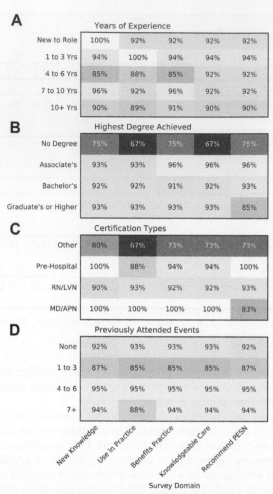

Fig. 2. Positive responses stratified by demographics of (*A*) years of experience, (*B*) highest degree achieved, (*C*) clinical certifications, and (*D*) previously attended events.

negative trend toward PESN providing benefits to clinical practice (75% positive, *P* = .235), and recommendation of PESN events to colleagues was also shown in participants with no college degree (75% positive, *P* = .096). Participants with no college degree significantly responded with a smaller proportion of positive responses with regard to if PESN provides them with more knowledgeable care (75% positive, *P* = .041). All other categories of degree achievement responded positively to the evaluation of PESN across all domains.

A similar trend across certification types with respondents who were classified as "other" certification giving fewer positive survey responses than other groups is shown in **Fig. 2**C. This was only appreciable as a trend that PESN provides new knowledge (80% positive, *P* = .120), benefits their practice (73% positive, *P* = .089), and provides them with more knowledgeable care (73% positive, *P* = .089). There were significantly fewer positive responses from the other certification group regarding that PESN provides information they can use in practice (67% positive, *P* = .018), and the recommendation of PESN events to others (73% positive, *P* = .036).

A very subtle decrease in positive responses was shown from survey participants who have previously attended 1 to 3 previous events (see **Fig. 2D**). This trend turns toward more positive responses as the respondents have attended 4 or more events. This could indicate participants who were unsatisfied after attending a few events and no longer came to PESN educational offerings. However, this could be a result of sampling error. Because sampling error could not be ruled out and the survey was not designed to evaluate this phenomenon, further study would be needed. The trends found within the demographic strata are likely unaffected by the missing responses because most missing responses were from RNs and prehospital providers and adding in the missing responses as positive responses only strengthens the trends.

The overall proportion among all questions and all responses showed that the vast majority of respondents (91.1%) had positive agreement that PESN and the education events are beneficial (n = 154). Historically, the average yearly attendance at PESN events has been increasing (**Fig. 3**). Although not statistically significant (R^2 = 0.44, P = .10), there is a positive trend that if continued by an increase of 5 participants per event, the average will achieve statistical significance within 1 year.

LIMITATIONS

The explanation of the online survey and paper survey were not designed to be of equal time or emphasis, so this may have contributed to the difference in response rate seen in our dataset. There is a possibility that a person could give duplicated responses to a survey, but this is expected to be a very unlikely event. The survey tool used was not validated, as there is not any widely used tool for our specific measurement goal. As this is self-assessment, voluntary survey of a convenience sample, the dataset is prone to all bias that accompanies such a model. Incomplete surveys with missing responses could have affected the data analysis.

DISCUSSION

Respondents who were classified as "other" certification tended to provide more negative survey responses than other groups. This could be because the educational events may not have been applicable to their particular role/profession. Further study for "other" certifications could help clarify this trend.

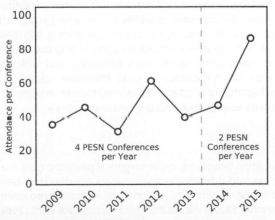

Fig. 3. Yearly attendance per PESN conference.

Barriers to outreach and education efforts can occur. One of the barriers to this education and outreach program included having enough staff available for the extra time needed to provide outreach education in addition to other ongoing patient care responsibilities. Allowing bedside staff time away from caring for patients in the busy health care environment to attend continuing education events was another barrier that was identified. For example, paramedics and EMTs were not able to attend educational events because of the need to have enough staff to cover 911 calls.

Competing educational events or conferences occurring around the same time as PESN educational events was another barrier to participation and attendance at PESN educational offerings. There were also other educational conferences specific to prehospital care and EMT and paramedic roles that they were required to attend that accounted for most of their allotted time for education and training. Therefore, participation of paramedics and EMTs was lower than for other health care providers.

A decision was made to increase PESN outreach and educational efforts to help address these barriers and increase outreach efforts. Average attendance at educational events at the beginning of this program was 35.75 participants. A substantial increase in attendance at PESN educational events occurred when PESN expanded its outreach efforts by offering educational events to participants outside the local PESN affiliates and opened it up to the community. Additional PESN outreach staff also helped to increase the number of people attending these events. A CNS was added to the PESN program in 2011 to help increase PESN education and outreach activities. A paramedic was also added to the PESN program in 2013 to help support the EMS community and further enhance outreach efforts. Attendance at PESN educational offerings increased from an average of 35.75 participants in the beginning of the program to an average attendance up to 86.5 at educational events in 2016 (see **Fig. 3**).

This education and outreach program can serve as a model for other health care facilities that wish to provide education and outreach to rural areas and the community. This program model can be used by other health care facilities and tailored to address specific types of diseases in different patient populations. For example, outreach education programs similar to this could be developed for adult asthma, diabetes, and other diseases and could be beneficial to those populations. Other types of education and outreach programs can have a positive impact at local and regional levels by addressing the educational needs of health care workers who provide care in the community.

This project focused on the educational outreach program, but a secondary outcome was to reduce nonemergent transfers from nonpediatric facilities and to improve quality of care for pediatric patients in the emergency setting. This unique program allows for a deeper sharing of knowledge among facilities. Providing specialty education has had a positive impact on establishing collaborative relationships and communication with local health care providers and will likely contribute to improved patient care and a reduction of cost. Proactive education will likely reduce unnecessary costs to patients and facilities related to mismanagement of pediatric patients and reduce cost associated with unnecessary transfers.

SUMMARY

Outreach and education programs on emergency pediatric care can have a positive impact by identifying and addressing the educational needs of health care workers who provide care in the community and in rural areas. Based on the results of this self-assessment survey study, we found that most respondents reported this education and outreach program provided new knowledge about pediatric emergency care and was beneficial to their clinical practice. Most participants also reported they planned to use the information they learned in their clinical practice and would recommend this education and outreach program to their colleagues. Outreach and education programs can address the educational needs of health care workers and have positive impact at local and regional levels.

REFERENCES

1. American College of Surgeons, Committee on Trauma. Resources for optimal care of the injured patient. 6th edition. Chicago (IL): American College of Surgeons; 2014. p. 134–8.
2. Kelley-Quon LI, Crowley MA, Applebaum H, et al. Academic-community partnerships improve outcomes in pediatric trauma care. J Pediatr Surg 2015;50: 1032–6.
3. Sumeet VJ, Castigliano MB, Cooney RN. Trauma transfers to a rural level 1 center: a retrospective cohort study. J Trauma Management Outcomes 2016;10:1.
4. Goldstein SD, Van Arendonk K, Aboagye JK, et al. Secondary overtriage in pediatric trauma: can unnecessary patient transfers be avoided? J Pediatr Surg 2015; 50(6):1028–31.
5. Committee on Pediatric Emergency Medicine. The role of the pediatrician in rural emergency medical services for children. Pediatrics 2012;130:978–82. Available at: http://pediatrics.aappublications.org/content/130/5/978.full.html. Accessed August 14, 2014.
6. Curran V, Rourke L, Snow P. A framework for enhancing continuing medical education for rural physicians: a summary of the literature. Med Teach 2010; 32(11):e501–8.
7. Garcia EA, Likourezos A, Ramsay C, et al. Evaluation of emergency medicine community educational program. West J Emerg Med 2010;11(5):416–8.
8. Curran JA, Murphy AL, Sinclair D, et al. Factors influencing rural and urban emergency clinicians' participation in an online knowledge exchange intervention. Rural Remote Health 2013;13(1):2175. Available at: http://www.rrh.org.au. Accessed February 23, 2015.
9. Policicchio NB, Nelson B, Duffy S. Bringing evidence-based continuing education on asthma to nurses. Clin Nurse Specialist 2011;25(3):125–32.
10. High K, Yeatman J. The development of an educational outreach program by one aeromedical service. J Emerg Nurs 1997;23(3):256–8.
11. Drury T, Zacharias S. Integrating nursing education into a trauma outreach program. Int J Trauma Nurs 1997;3(3):83–7.
12. Paulson DJ. A rural outreach program for emergency nurses. J Emerg Nurs 1996; 22:125–30.
13. Harris PA, Taylor R, Thielke R, et al. Research electronic data capture (REDCap): a metadata-driven methodology and workflow process for providing translational research informatics support. J Biomed Inform 2009;42(2):377–81.

APPENDIX 1: PEDIATRIC EMERGENCY SERVICES NETWORK (PESN) AND TRAUMA SERVICES EDUCATION EVALUATION TOOL

Confidential

Pediatric Emergency Services Network (PESN) & Trauma Services Education Evaluation Tool

The PESN mission is to enhance and improve emergency care of pediatric patients by providing regular pediatric emergency and pediatric trauma education to the community and emergency personnel.

Please complete the survey below to help us evaluate the PESN educational offering that you most recently attended.

1   Date of PESN educational event that you most recently
    attended   _____
                                                                (Please supply the date of the education event you
                                                                attended)

2   Have you previously submitted a paper version of this   ○ Yes
    survey for the event date entered above?   ○ No

3   Gender   ○ Male
                                                                ○ Female

4   Ethnicity   ○ Hispanic or Latino
                                                                ○ Not Hispanic or Latino

5   Race (check all that apply)   ☐ American Indian or Alaska Native
                                                                ☐ Asian
                                                                ☐ Black or African American
                                                                ☐ Native Hawaiian or Other Pacific Islander
                                                                ☐ White
                                                                ☐ Other

    If Other is selected please list: _____

6   How long have you worked as a healthcare provider?

    ○ New to my role   ○ 1 to 3 years   ○ 4 to 6 years   ○ 7 to 10 years   ○ More than 10 years

7   What is the highest level of education you have   ○ High school or GED
    attained?   ○ Some college, no degree
                                                                ○ Associate's degree
                                                                ○ Bachelor's degree
                                                                ○ Graduate or professional degree
                                                                ○ Doctorate

8   What board certifications or licensures do you   ☐ None
    currently hold? (check all that apply)   ☐ EMT - Basic
                                                                ☐ EMT - Paramedic / Licensed Paramedic
                                                                ☐ RT
                                                                ☐ RN
                                                                ☐ LVN
                                                                ☐ APN
                                                                ☐ PA
                                                                ☐ MD / DO
                                                                ☐ Other, Not Listed

    Please list other board certifications or licensures   _____
    you currently hold.

9   How many PESN Education Events have your attended in the past?

    ○ None   ○ 1 to 3   ○ 4 to 6   ○ 7 to 9   ○ Greater than 10

*Survey continued on other side / next page *

REDCap

In regards to the PESN training you have just attended, please rank your agreement with the following statements.

	Strongly Disagree	Disagree	Neutral	Agree	Strongly Agree
10 This educational event provided me with new knowledge about pediatric emergency care.	O	O	O	O	O
11 I plan to use the information I learned at this educational event in my clinical practice.	O	O	O	O	O

In regards to PESN as a whole please rank your agreement with the following statements.

	Strongly Disagree	Disagree	Neutral	Agree	Strongly Agree
12 The education that PESN provides benefits my clinical practice.	O	O	O	O	O
13 I feel more knowledgeable about providing pediatric emergency care because of the education I have received from PESN.	O	O	O	O	O
14 I would recommend PESN events to my colleagues.	O	O	O	O	O

* This concludes the survey *

REDCap

Courtesy of UT Southwestern, REDCap System, Dallas, TX; with permission.

Pediatric Mild Traumatic Brain Injury and Population Health

An Introduction for Nursing Care Providers

Michelle Borzik Goreth, MSN, RN-BC, CPNP-AC, CCRN-P, CTRN, CPEN, TCRN

KEYWORDS

- Pediatric mild traumatic brain injury • Concussion • Population health
- Health-related quality of life • Health disparities • Pediatric trauma

KEY POINTS

- Prevention of mild traumatic brain injury is essential to improve population health.
- Identification of health disparities in pediatric mild traumatic brain injury is essential to minimize impact of injury.
- Improving health-related quality of life after pediatric mild traumatic brain injury is essential to reduce lifetime economic burden.

TRAUMATIC BRAIN INJURY IN THE UNITED STATES

Injury is the leading cause of mortality in the United States in ages 1 to 44.[1] Traumatic brain injury (TBI), specifically, is a major contributor to population death and disability, accounting for 30% of all traumatic deaths. Caused by a bump, jolt, blow, penetrating, or impulsive trauma to the head, TBI results in disruption of normal neurologic function of the brain, producing symptoms ranging from mild to severe. Rates of TBI have continued to grow over the last several decades, with most recent estimates from the Centers for Disease Control and Prevention reporting approximately 2.5 million cases per year from emergency department (ED) visits, hospitalizations, and deaths. Rising rates of TBI have direct impact on population health and increase the burden on the US economy and health system. The true extent of population health impact as a result of TBI is unknown because of underestimation of incidence; underreporting of

Disclosure Statement: The author has nothing to disclose.
Division of Pediatric Surgery, Department of Surgery, University of Mississippi Medical Center, 2500 North State Street, Jackson, MS 39216, USA
E-mail address: dmgoreth@umc.edu

mild injuries; and the potential for nonreversible, chronic health effects that can continue to occur across the lifespan. Considering these uncertainties, TBI prevention is of national importance and is recognized as one of the most preventable causes of injury, death, and disability.[1]

Children are more susceptible than adults to TBI. Differences in pediatric anatomy and physiology, such as a disproportionally large head compared with body size, lack of fusion of skull bones, immature neurologic function, and inability to recognize or avoid injury because of age/developmental stage predisposes children to higher risk of injury.[1,2] In addition to pathophysiologic and developmental differences, health disparities exist in pediatric trauma care that further increase risk of injury and impact treatment and recovery from TBI. While general access to health care has improved over the last decade, children with Medicaid or Child Health Insurance Program coverage may not obtain care as soon as desired and receive lower quality of care, especially in southern states.[3] National efforts to reduce general disparities in minority children and those with lower socioeconomic status have been unsuccessful and remain unchanged.[3,4]

Disparities specific to pediatric trauma care include limited numbers of pediatric trauma centers, pediatric surgeons, and pediatric specialists to support trauma care, and significant health inequities that exist among African American children.[5] African American children have a higher prevalence of comorbidities before injury compared with other ethnicities and have longer lengths of hospital stay, functional outcomes that are worse, and higher need for inpatient rehabilitation after all types of trauma care.[6] Additional disparities have been suggested in health care provider bias and cultural differences in the care of African American children with TBI because they are more likely to be cared for by a resident physician and less likely to be hospitalized or receive follow-up care. Mortality after TBI has also been reported higher among African American children (5.3%) compared with white children (2.2%).[4,7]

Despite inequities in care, higher risks, and increasing incidence, children with TBI sustain less severe injuries and have higher survival rates compared with adults.[1,8,9] Children who have a TBI, therefore, carry a higher overall burden on society. Loss of productivity has to be weighed for the parents of the injured child and across the lifespan of the child with TBI, considering that chronic effects may not develop or be recognized until the child ages. Chronic health effects may vary in severity and manifest themselves either as a single entity or exist in combination as an impairment, disruption in functional status, disability, or reduction in health-related quality of life (HRQOL).[1] Efforts to prevent injuries that result in pediatric TBI, improve quality of care and recovery after injury, and reduce associated disparities in pediatric trauma care are paramount to lower future health care costs, improve societal productivity, and enhance population health.

IMPACT OF PEDIATRIC TRAUMATIC BRAIN INJURY ON THE HEALTH SYSTEM

Overall increase in incidence of TBI has been linked to increase in ED visits, as TBI-related hospitalizations have essentially remained stable and TBI-related deaths have decreased slightly. In 2009 to 2010, an average of 11.9 million injury-related ED visits occurred involving children and adolescents ages 0 to 18 years.[8,9] Publicly funded insurance coverage (41.7%), Medicaid or Child Health Insurance Program, and no insurance coverage (8.6%) comprised expected payor sources in more than half the ED visits. Mechanisms of injuries for all injury-related ED visits were highest for falls and striking against or being struck by an object or persons in males and females. Visits for all unintentional injuries were noted to be highest in males across all age groups with non-Hispanic black males having the highest rate of all injury-related visits compared with all races and ethnicities in ages 5 to 18 years.[10]

TBI from all mechanisms of injury results in approximately 500,000 ED visits annually. Falls are the leading mechanism of TBI in children ages 0 to 14 years. For this age group, the Centers for Disease Control and Prevention reported 352,203 ED visits that occurred as a result of falls during 2009 to 2010. Ages 0 to 4 years had the highest occurrence, accounting for 72.8% of TBI-related ED visits in this age group. Mechanisms of injury for TBI-related visits in ages 5 to 14 years were highest for being struck by or against an object (34.9%) and falls (35.1%), accounting for 70% of TBI-related ED visits in ages 5 to 14 years.[10]

Overall rates of hospitalization in children decreased from 2001 to 2010, with significant decreases in hospitalizations in ages 5 to 14 years. During this time frame, rates of hospitalizations in ages 0 to 4 years decreased from 70.3 to 57.7 per 100,000 and in ages 5 to 14 years decreased by more than 50% from 54.4 to 23.1 per 100,000. Falls remain the leading cause of hospital admission because of TBI in children ages 0 to 14 years with higher rates in ages 0 to 4 years of age.[9] Medicaid insurance coverage, older child, and admission to a pediatric trauma center have been linked to increased length of hospital stay for children admitted to a hospital after TBI.[11] All pediatric TBI-related deaths have decreased to an average rate of 6.2 per 100,000 except in ages 0 to 4 years where rates increased to 4.3 per 100,000 compared with ages 5 to 14 years at 1.9 per 100,000.[8,9]

Treatment of injury at a designated trauma center has long been identified to improve injury-related morbidity and mortality and optimize outcomes.[12] Over the last several decades, pediatric trauma centers have been established to support the unique needs of the pediatric trauma patient that may not be readily available in adult trauma systems, such as pediatric-trained specialist or appropriately sized equipment. Children treated for any mechanism of injury at pediatric trauma centers demonstrate improved outcomes, decreased length of hospital stay, lower mortality rates, and improved access to specialists and rehabilitation.[5] However, most children do not receive care at dedicated pediatric trauma centers, especially for less severe injuries, such as mild TBI. Education and development of appropriate guidelines for the treatment of injured children must be created and supported by triage systems to assist providers with guidance of transfer to definitive pediatric care.[12]

Despite the availability of pediatric trauma centers, approximately 17 million children do not have access to a pediatric trauma center within 60 minutes.[12] Children with lower levels of injury severity, such as mild TBI, may be admitted for evaluation and management at centers without available pediatric specialties. Providers at non-pediatric trauma centers, and pediatric trauma centers, must but be aware of social determinants and health disparities, or preventable entities that can affect pediatric trauma care, risk of injury, and impacts of ongoing management.

Low literacy and educational levels, racial disparities, lower incomes and socioeconomic status, high rates of crime and violence, poor housing conditions, high rates of public insurance coverage, significant disease comorbidities, and geographic distance from a single pediatric trauma care system may lead to poorer trauma outcomes and effect population health and their impacts vary by state.[3,6] With general increased risk of injury in children, accompanied by health disparities and inequalities in pediatric trauma care, societal burden after TBI in children produces significant strain on the US economy and health care system resulting in larger economic impacts from those with nonfatal injuries (not requiring hospitalization or resulting in death).[9]

SIGNIFICANCE OF TRAUMATIC BRAIN INJURY ON POPULATION HEALTH

In addition to ED visits, approximately 10 million primary care visits are related to injury annually, making injury one of the principal reasons people seek health care. National estimates report nearly 15,000 children will die and approximately 20,000 will develop permanent disabilities, most as a result of head injury.[5] Despite increasing national incidence and associated morbidity and mortality, most TBI in children is mild.[13] However mild, pediatric patients that sustain a mild traumatic brain injury may have immediate and long-term sequelae that are among the most frequent causes of interruption to normal child development.[10,11]

Early recognition, treatment, and evaluation of TBI and comorbidities that may prolong symptoms are essential to improve recovery and outcomes. Mild TBI comprises 80% to 90% of all pediatric TBI and may often be overlooked in the inpatient environment, especially in critical care units, for more severe, concomitant injuries or deemed less important because children may not have visible or external signs of injury.[14] Mild TBI, or concussion, is defined by any alteration in mental status after direct or impulsive traumatic impact to the head and does not have to occur with loss of consciousness.[13] Recent studies suggest that 85% of pediatric mild TBI occurs without the loss of consciousness. In addition, diagnostic imaging used in evaluation of injury, such as computerized tomography of the head, may be negative for structural injury, which may make it difficult to identify pediatric mild TBI, especially in younger children, and thus making thorough and ongoing neurologic and cognitive assessment/evaluation essential.[15]

Health effects occurring after TBI may be categorized by clinical manifestation: physical, cognitive, behavioral/emotional, and sleep-related symptoms. Symptoms may be present in one or more categories at varying time frames and severity after injury. When lasting greater than 1 month, symptoms may be collectively termed postconcussive syndrome. In addition, psychological or neurologic conditions, such as posttraumatic stress syndrome, depression, or posttraumatic epilepsy, may develop after TBI, increasing burden of injury with additional illness and complexity of care. Children with premorbid behavioral, emotional, or physical illnesses, especially preexisting headaches, may also have worsened exacerbation of premorbid disorders and prolonged postconcussive symptoms that impact quality of life and return of function after TBI.[16,17]

Mild TBI postconcussive symptoms are difficult to evaluate. In adults, resolution of symptoms in mild TBI is expected between 7 and 10 days in 80% to 90% of the adult population.[1] However, children and adolescents may take longer for symptom resolution.[16] Incidence of postconcussive symptoms is often underestimated in children because of underreporting or failure to seek medical care after mild injuries, inability to recognize symptoms in younger or nonverbal children, or avoidance of reporting in such cases as abuse. Postconcussive symptoms may be temporary or permanent and are thought to be present even after mild TBI in an estimated 145,000 children age 0 to 19 years.[1] Children with postconcussive symptoms are at risk for further impairments in physical, psychological, and social functioning that can effect ongoing developmental processes related to learning, social interaction, and emotional awareness, leading to functional limitation or disability and reduced quality of life for the child and the family.[16,18]

HEALTH-RELATED QUALITY OF LIFE

HRQOL is a concept that attempts to identify all aspects of a disease or illness process that may affect a person's physical, mental, or social well-being.[16] HRQOL in children is measured based on physical function, cognitive function, emotional function, social function, school function, and psychosocial function. Evaluation of HRQOL may differ among parents and their children because it is a self-reported entity. Although minimal research has been performed to evaluate HRQOL after pediatric TBI, general themes support that children with more severe injuries have been identified as having lower HRQOL compared to those with mild TBI and presence of pre-existing psychosocial conditions is associated with significant reduction in all aspects of HRQOL, regardless of the severity of injury.[16–19]

Several keys risk factors have been identified for lower HRQOL after mild TBI in children. Preinjury behavioral or school problems, lower socioeconomic status and lower income, Medicaid or lack of insurance coverage, lower level of parental education, Hispanic ethnicity, older age at time of injury, single parent home, and family dysfunction have been identified as showing poorer HRQOL post-TBI. Larger number of physical and cognitive postconcussive symptoms has also been shown to be associated with lower psychosocial HRQOL. In addition to physical and cognitive symptoms that impact general daily function, caregivers who reported unmet needs or whose children did not receive adequate services have been identified as having a lower HRQOL.[16–19]

Cognitive dysfunction is one of the most concerning symptoms for parents. After somatic symptoms, poor concentration or memory deficits are the most reportable concerns.[18] Cognitive dysfunction impacts all aspects of HRQOL. Lapses in attention or memory produce academic difficulties and have potential to increase risk of further injury. Slower cognitive abilities or processing might also impact peer-social interactions by slower communication or inability to have abstract thought, leading to difficulties with social interaction and adjustment. Pre-existing psychosocial problems may also further decrease social functioning. Difficulties with poor self-esteem, loneliness, maladjustment, or social isolation may intensify the lack of emotional control and aggressive behaviors after injury, leading to difficulties with ongoing development of social skills and potential loss of productivity caused by inability to adjust, problem solve, or interact with others. In addition, such conditions as family dysfunction, permissive parenting, and lack of family resources have also been identified as risk factors that impact social function and decrease HRQOL after pediatric TBI.[20]

Family burden is increased after TBI and is worse in more severe injuries. Those children with higher behavioral and functional problems have higher reported burdens on families, specifically when emotional or social function is impacted. In addition to stress from injury, financial burden may add to poorer HRQOL because of medical costs or loss of parental productivity from multiple medical appointments. Perceived increase in caregiver burden has been identified when the child's needs are unmet. Children with lower severity of TBI have the highest rates of unmet needs, especially during the first year after injury. Unmet needs may be caused by lack of access to care, such as rehabilitation, or lack of insurance coverage for needed services. Children with Medicaid and those from dysfunctional families are at higher risk for inadequate services or referrals.[21] Many children with TBI may also require mental health services, which may be partially or not covered under insurance plans.[22] Slomine and colleagues[21] suggest that poor outcomes in families with lower socioeconomic status and poorer family function may actually be related to inadequate receipt of early post–acute care services designed to identify or resolve injury-related problems.

Efforts to identify at-risk children after pediatric mild TBI can assist in early implementation of support services to reduce overall burden of injury and improve HRQOL. Impact of TBI on the family and caregiver can also effect HRQOL. Improvement is needed to identify the family at-risk to assist in providing early postinjury support, improve access to services, and reduce family or caregiver burden after pediatric mild TBI to reduce long-term impact on population health and economic strain.

REDUCING IMPACTS OF MILD TRAUMATIC BRAIN INJURY DURING HOSPITALIZATION

Currently, no standard accepted guidelines exist for inpatient or outpatient management of pediatric mild TBI but early physical and cognitive rest along with prevention of secondary injury are the mainstays of therapy.[2] In inpatient care, this can often be difficult to achieve, especially in the intensive care environment, where frequent or hourly neurologic assessments of any person with TBI is the standard of care.[23] Nursing care should promote physical and cognitive rest with low-stimulation environments. Planned interventions may include noise-reduction strategies, restricted visitation, dimming room light and computer displays, and clustering of care. Staff, patients, and families should be encouraged to minimize use of music or other devices emitting noise and limit computer, television, telephone, or video screen time. Patient and families should be incorporated in care planning and provided education on mild TBI and treatment plans, including injury prevention education throughout hospitalization.

Development of TBI screening protocols may assist in early identification of cognitive deficits or need for rehabilitation care because children with mild TBI may not have visible, external injury. Use of occupational, physical, and speech therapies and early intervention specialists are useful resources to assist in early and ongoing screenings for cognitive and physical deficits. Monitoring psychosocial impact after trauma can assist in identification of ineffective coping or posttraumatic stress. School-related support or services can assist in bridging return to academic activities for those with cognitive impairments. Although race and gender disparities may not be easily altered, inpatient screening and providing interventions for comorbidities and lack of insurance coverage to facilitate follow-up care before discharge directly addresses known disparities in pediatric trauma care. Incorporating dedicated case management and social services support for trauma care can enhance patient insurance coverage and ensure follow-up care and monitoring. Lastly, development of institutional guidelines and transfer plans help support provider decision making when referral to pediatric trauma specialty care may be indicated.

THE CARE PROVIDER'S ROLE IN PEDIATRIC TRAUMATIC BRAIN INJURY

Initial interactions between care providers and children with TBI are usually in the face of acute injury. The primary role of medical and nursing care teams is to provide stabilization, treatment, and identify early impairments that may necessitate rehabilitation. Developing an understanding of TBI and its impacts from injury through rehabilitation is crucial. This begins with implementing basic mild TBI care, such as physical and cognitive rest, and becoming aware of social determinants of health and health inequities that may exist in the care of pediatric trauma patients. Although recent guidelines have been published for the care of pediatric severe TBI injuries, lack of general consensus or guidelines for care of pediatric mild TBI have yet to be published.[1] Therefore, all providers must stay acutely aware of emerging research and identify at-risk populations to enhance care, improve outcomes and HRQOL, and reduce overall burden to population health caused by TBI.

Advanced practice nursing providers can also assist in decreasing the gap in determining epidemiology and consequences of pediatric TBI by participating in surveillance activities that address more accurate documentation of mechanisms of injury; measures of HRQOL such as cognitive, emotional/behavioral, and social effects of injury; and disabilities to obtain more accurate evaluation of long-term complications from TBI. Surveillance also assists in identifying areas to improve injury prevention efforts, increase access to care, develop support systems, reduce health disparities and inequalities, and leads to policy development that can drive improvement in outcomes after TBI.

The greatest impact in reducing impact from TBI can be made by focusing efforts to prevent injuries. Despite health inequities and disparities, no one is immune to trauma and it can affect individuals without regard to geographic location, socioeconomic status, race/ethnicity, health status, or any other demographic. National injury prevention initiatives should focus on safety measures to prevent injuries caused by falls and motor vehicle collisions, the leading mechanisms of injury among children in the United States.[1]

Introduction of fall prevention and safety should occur in the form of anticipatory guidance during patient encounters, from birth through teenage years, but especially in ages 0 to 4 years where falls are greatest. Counseling and education should be provided on safe sleeping habits and developmental abilities, appropriate activities by age, importance of adult supervision, or specific safety equipment for such activities as helmet use with bicycle riding. Injury from motor vehicle collision can occur in vehicle occupants and pedestrian or cyclists that are bystanders. In children, efforts to promote appropriate car safety restraint use is the single most important component of injury reduction. Education during any patient encounter, but especially at well-child checks, is an optimal time to reinforce car safety restraint use.[24] Nurses should engage in community injury prevention and outreach efforts, such as health fairs, where safety education information is disseminated to larger groups and may have greater impact on injury reduction and improvement in population health.

Opportunities to promote injury prevention may also exist outside the clinical arena. Participation in research or serving on local, regional, state, and national committees to evaluate injury patterns and develop injury prevention recommendations for communities or businesses are direct ways to reduce injuries. Examples include development of new care guidelines or tools for providers; recommendations for design of newer safety innovations in air bags or restraint systems; improvement in infrastructure, such as increasing traffic lights or building sidewalks in urban areas where motor vehicles are more prevalent; or development of booster restraint laws in older children.[24] To create injury prevention strategies that are effective, enhanced TBI surveillance systems are needed to further research efforts that enhance understanding of TBI prevalence and its long-term impacts.[1]

SUMMARY

TBI is the leading cause of death and disability in the United States and has significant impact on population health. Prevalence of TBI has increased in children over the last several decades, especially in ages 0 to 4 years, placing increased strain on the health system and economy. Additional lifetime costs and economic burden are caused by low mortality rates in children with TBI. With increased survival, children carry higher rates of long-term or chronic effects from impairments and disabilities. Early recognition of TBI in outpatient and inpatient care is essential for ongoing evaluation and management of acute symptoms and reduction of chronic health effects and disabilities that may be sustained after TBI. Providing early interventions to manage acute and postconcussive symptoms in mild TBI can minimize adverse events that reduce HRQOL for the injured child and their family. Ensuring health insurance coverage, improving access to pediatric trauma care specialists, and providing ongoing monitoring during hospitalization and postdischarge to meet rehabilitation needs enhances TBI outcomes and combats health inequities. Despite the presence of health disparities, especially in African American children, all children are at increased risk for TBI. Key efforts to minimize impact of TBI on population health should focus on injury prevention strategies and elimination of health disparities in at-risk populations.

REFERENCES

1. Centers for Disease Control. Report to Congress on traumatic brain injury in the United States: epidemiology and rehabilitation. Atlanta (GA): National Center for Injury Prevention and Control; Division of Unintentional Injury Prevention; 2015. Available at: http://www.cdc.gov/traumaticbraininjury/pdf/ tbi_report_to_congress_epi_ and_rehab-a.pdf. Accessed July 21, 2016.

2. Mason CM. Mild traumatic brain injury in children. Pediatr Nurs 2013;39(6): 267–72, 282.

3. Agency for Healthcare Research and Quality. 2014 National healthcare and quality disparities report; AHRQ Pub. No. 15–0007. 2015. Available at: http://www. ahrq.gov/sites/default/files/wysiwyg/research/findings/nhqrdr/nhqdr14/2014nhqdr. pdf. Accessed July 20, 2016.

4. Brown RL. Epidemiology of injury and the impact of health disparities. Curr Opin Pediatr 2009;22:321–5.

5. Petrosyan M, Guner YS, Enami CN, et al. Disparities in the delivery of pediatric trauma care. J Trauma 2009;67(2 Suppl):S114–9.

6. Haider AH, Efron DT, Haut ER, et al. Black children experience worse clinical and functional outcomes after traumatic brain injury: an analysis of the national pediatric trauma registry. J Trauma 2007;62(5):1259–63.

7. Falcone RA, Martin C, Brown RL, et al. Despite overall low pediatric head injury mortality, disparities exist between races. J Pediatr Surg 2008;43(10):1858–64.

8. Centers for Disease Control. Rates of TBI-related deaths by age group-United States 2001-2010. 2016. Available at: http://www.cdc.gov/traumaticbraininjury/ data/rates_deaths_byage.html. Accessed July 6, 2016.

9. Centers for Disease Control. Rates of TBI-related hospitalizations by age group-United States 2001-2010. 2016. Available at: http://www.cdc.gov/traumaticbrain injury/data/rates_hosp_byage.html. Accessed July 6, 2016.

10. Albert M, McCaig LF. Injury-related emergency department visits by children and adolescents: United States, 2009–2010. NCHS Data Brief No. 150. Atlanta (GA): National Center for Injury Prevention and Control; Division of Unintentional Injury Prevention; 2014. Available at: http://www.cdc.gov/nchs/data/databriefs/db150. pdf. Accessed July 8, 2016.

11. Schneier AJ, Shields BJ, Grim-Hostetler S, et al. Incidence of pediatric traumatic brain injury and associated hospital resource utilization in the United States. Pediatrics 2006;118(2):483–92.

12. Carr BG, Nance ML. Access to pediatric trauma care: alignment of providers and health systems. Curr Opin Pediatr 2010;22(3):326–31.

13. Yeates KO. Mild traumatic brain injury and postconcussive symptoms in children and adolescents. J Int Neuropsychol Soc 2010;16(6):953–60.

14. Struder M, Simonetti BG, Joeris A, et al. Post-concussive symptoms and neuropsychological performance in the post-acute period following pediatric mild traumatic brain injury. J Int Neuropsychol Soc 2014;20(10):982–93.

15. Lee LK, Monroe D, Bachman MC, et al. Isolated loss of consciousness in children with minor blunt head trauma. JAMA Pediatr 2014;168(9):837–43.
16. Fineblit S, Selci E, Loewen H, et al. Health-related quality of life after pediatric mild traumatic brain injury/concussion: a systematic review. J Neurotrauma 2016;33:1–8.
17. McCarthy ML, MacKenzie EJ, Durbin DR, et al. Health-related quality of life during the first year after traumatic brain injury. Arch Pediatr Adolesc Med 2006; 160(3):252–60.
18. Moran LM, Taylor HG, Rusin J, et al. Quality of life in pediatric mild traumatic brain injury and its relationship to postconcussive symptoms. J Pediatr Psychol 2012; 37(7):736–44.
19. Piper P, Garvan C. Health-related quality-of-life in the first year following a childhood concussion. Brain Inj 2014;28(1):105–13.
20. Rosema S, Crowe L, Anderson V. Social function in children and adolescents after traumatic brain injury: a systematic review 1989-2011. J Neurotrauma 2012;29(7): 1277–91.
21. Slomine BS, McCarthy ML, Ding R, et al. Health care utilization and needs after pediatric traumatic brain injury. Pediatrics 2006;117(4):e663–74.
22. Aitken ME, McCarthy ML, Slomine BS. Family burden after traumatic brain injury in children. Pediatrics 2009;123(1):199–206.
23. American Association of Neuroscience Nurses and Association of Rehabilitation Nurses. Care of the patient with mild traumatic brain injury. 2011. Available at: http://www.rehabnurse.org/uploads/files/cpgmtbi.pdf. Accessed July 24, 2016.
24. Dewan MC, Mummareddy M, Wellons JC, et al. Epidemiology of global pediatric traumatic brain injury: Qualitative review. World Neurosurgery 2016;91:497–509.

When Nursing Assertion Stops

A Qualitative Study to Examine the Cultural Barriers Involved in Escalation of Care in a Pediatric Hospital

Jodi Thrasher, MSN, RN, CFNP[a],*, Heidi McNeely, MSN, RN, PCNS-BC[a],
Bonnie Adrian, PhD, RN[b]

KEYWORDS

- Code reduction • Rapid response teams • Nurse perception • Code barriers
- Rapid response team barriers • Pediatric nursing

KEY POINTS

- Nurses regarded rapid response team (RRT) calls as requests for a provider-to-provider consult such that initiation ought to be by the provider, not the nurse.
- RRT calls that do not lead to transfer of the patient to an ICU may be viewed as false alarms indicative of a failure of nursing clinical expertise.
- Nurses described physicians as wanting to try interventions on the floor first before calling an RRT, requiring excessive nursing time not appropriate to the medicine unit setting and contributing to delays in escalation of care.
- Nurses reported having strong assertion skills yet described clinical experiences in which "assertion" consisted of time spent attempting to convince physicians to call an RRT rather than calling the RRT themselves.

BACKGROUND

Reducing codes outside of ICUs has been a national and international focus in recent years. The term, code reduction, refers to clinical efforts to reduce the incidence of pulmonary and/or cardiac arrest that necessitates life-saving resuscitation. Code reduction involves a complex set of clinical activities, including early detection of signs and symptoms, communication among nursing and medical providers, and performance of clinical interventions to treat a patient's deterioration. Ideally,

---

The authors have nothing to disclose.
[a] Inpatient Medical Unit, Children's Hospital Colorado, 13123 East 16th Avenue, B485, Aurora, CO 80045, USA; [b] Clinical Informatics, University of Colorado Health, 12401 East 17th Avenue, Aurora, CO 80045, USA
* Corresponding author.
E-mail address: jodi.thrasher@childrenscolorado.org

cardiopulmonary arrest would never occur on inpatient medical or surgical units because patients at risk of deterioration would be identified early and transferred to an ICU. Although rare, codes sometimes occur on the inpatient units. Many hospitals have implemented rapid response programs, known as RRTs or medical emergency teams, as an avenue for staff to escalate patient care needs. Rapid response program investments have not produced the level of reduction for code events that hospitals anticipated. This has generated interest in understanding barriers to success. The Medical Early Response Intervention and Therapy trial[1] found that rapid response system activation only occurred 30% of the time when clinical criteria were met in 250 cardiac arrests. A systematic review[2] demonstrated that failure to rescue rates vary between 8% to 16.9% and contributing causes may include failure to recognize clinical deterioration, failure to escalate, and failure to activate RRTs.

Nurses play a critical role in rapid response through identification of patient deterioration and communication of clinical changes. Nurses are trained to identify subtle changes and recognize signs of deterioration in the patient's condition.[3–6] Shearer and colleagues[7] found that failures in the system were most often not due to problems with recognition but instead due to challenges inherent in hospital cultures and clinical hierarchies. Roberts and colleagues[8] reported that nurses with lower self-efficacy often need consultation with another nurse to validate their concerns prior to activating an RRT, whereas the presence of self-efficacy can assist in overcoming challenges in hospital hierarchies.

Interdisciplinary hierarchies complicate nursing communication.[9] Some barriers to activating RRTs identified in the literature[5,8] include situations when nurses thought their patient was at risk but were uncomfortable going up the chain of command to preserve the relationship within the team. Nurses often solicit feedback and partner with other nurses to overcome this hierarchy.[8] Shearer and colleagues[7] found that RRTs may not be activated "because of the poor sensitivity and specificity of the activation criteria." A similar finding by Braaten revealed that clinicians require "justification" for RRT activation "to avoid false alarms."[6] Mathematical analysis of rapid response activation criteria's predictive sensitivity and specificity reveals that "33 calls would be needed to prevent one unplanned ICU transfer, cardiac arrest, or death. Nurses' attempts to minimize false-positive calls may help explain the low call rates for patients meeting RRT criteria."[10]

In previous studies[4,5,11] nurses were often alerted to deteriorating clinical condition because they perceived that something was wrong or they were "concerned about the patient." This feeling of concern was cited as more important than the measurement of vital signs.[11] Nurses have to synthesize all the evidence and determine when to call a provider or RRT. A nurse's decision to call for help was influenced by the ability to demonstrate confidence in knowledge of situations, strength of evidence of clinical deterioration, and the ability to balance and manage situations with the available resources.[11] Minick and Harvey[4] found that when nurses recognized small changes in a patient's condition they are more successful in getting physicians to act if they could describe these changes clearly when lacking objective data. Early warning score systems have allowed nurses to have tools for more objective reporting.[12,13] Nurses present evidence of and describe deterioration using intuitive knowing and objective findings.[12] In addition, nurses have to package the communication to persuade doctors to assess the patient.[11,12] If the doctor is not persuaded, this can result in a failure where the patient is not evaluated.[11] There needs to be more effort in understanding individual and bedside cultural issues that may prevent staff from activating an RRT and preventing a code event.

OBJECTIVE

The purpose of the current study is to evaluate nurses' perceptions of barriers to early clinical intervention for code reduction on the inpatient medical unit at a free-standing pediatric academic medical center. This research originated from the stated needs of the unit's advanced practice nurses (APNs), who serve as clinical experts for the unit and expressed frustration with the resistance of code rates to decline in response to positive changes made on the unit. Formalization of the RRT program in the organization occurred in 2007. Initially, the hospital participated in the Children's Hospital Association collaborative work on code reduction in 2007 to 2008. This led to many interventions, including interdisciplinary code simulations, case review, radar rounds, and formalization of the RRT program. Code simulations involve an interdisciplinary team in either a high-fidelity laboratory setting or in a low-fidelity unit-based setting. These simulations are intended to meet the goals of facilitating team collaboration and enhancing team communication while identifying educational gaps. Case reviews are constructed by the APNs based on actual scenarios that occurred on the inpatient medical unit. Radar rounds are a daily process where the charge nurse and senior provider talk at the start of each shift to identify patients who may have the potential to deteriorate. This allows for the interdisciplinary team to have a heightened awareness about patients on the unit. The inpatient medical unit has conducted case reviews of all of its codes since 2007. Aggregated data from the unit's code case reviews suggest that nurses perform well at early identification of troubling signs and symptoms yet sometimes fail to escalate in a timely, effective manner. Assertion training occurred in early 2012 within the organization to address escalation of care situations and equip staff with communication tools. Even with all these efforts focused on increasing awareness and reducing barriers, unit leaders suspected that there may be other unidentified barriers in the workplace culture that prevent nurses from escalating their concerns for clinical deterioration. This study sought to identify such barriers.

DESIGN, DATA COLLECTION, AND PARTICIPANTS

This study, approved by the Colorado Multiple Institutional Review Board, uses a qualitative design with convenience sampling. In-depth nurse interviews elicited detailed narratives of nurses' experiences with successful and unsuccessful management of clinical deterioration. In addition, nurses were invited to share their perceptions of barriers to reducing the incidence of code blue events outside the ICUs.

Participants from the inpatient medical unit were recruited via e-mails, flyers, and verbal invitations to participate. All recruitment activities specified that participation was voluntary and open to any nurse on the inpatient medical unit who had one or both of the following types of nursing experiences: (1) direct care of a patient whose clinical status deteriorated to the point of code or (2) direct care of a patient who required an RRT activation. Ten nurses volunteered to participate and completed interviews of approximately 1 hour in length (**Table 1**).

Research on clinician missteps in cases of clinical deterioration involves inherent risks to study participants. In addition, the completeness and accuracy of study data are a risk in the event that study participants do not feel safe to speak forthrightly. The study team designed the protocol to include exceptionally rigorous steps to minimize risk of exposure to study participants and improve the completeness and accuracy of participants' interviews. Confidentiality of the participants was maintained by directing interested participants to the member of the research team who was not affiliated with the hospital. This researcher obtained consent and completed interviews at

Table 1 Nurse participant demographics		
Years of Registered Nursing Experience	Number of Registered Nurses	Role
<1	0	New-graduate RNs
<3	3	Staff RN
3–5	5	Staff RN
>5	1	Charge RN
>10	1	Charge RN
	N = 10	

a location of the participant's choosing. The consent process prior to the start of each interview included thorough review and discussion of the following added procedures to minimize risks of confidentiality: the interviewing researcher handled interview recordings and transcripts offsite, working with a professional transcriptionist, and removing identifiers during transcription and on transcript review. Due to the close nature of nursing professional relationships on the unit and unit leader knowledge of specific deterioration cases as a result of the unit's strong case review process, in some instances descriptions of individuals were redacted or altered to protect confidentiality. The research participant was given the opportunity to review his or her interview transcript after transcriptionist and interviewer deidentification efforts to ensure participant satisfaction with deidentification. Finally, the interviewer broke down all interview transcripts into segments, mixing interspersed segments from all 10 interviews together prior to sharing the data with the rest of the research team. Disaggregating interview transcript data provides additional confidentiality protection in that if a nurse is recognizable from her involvement in a case she described, unit leaders' identification of the nurse in that particular case does not allow them to associate other statements by the same nurse with her.

Each member of the study team reviewed the transcript data, leading to discussion of various themes beyond the scope of this article. The analytical themes that study team members agreed were most salient for advancing the literature on cultural barriers to reducing code blue events are presented.

SETTING

The research organization is a freestanding academic children's hospital with more than 486 beds in the Rocky Mountain region. The study took place on an inpatient medical unit consisting of 82 inpatient medical beds on 2 different floors of the hospital. The unit has 6 main provider teams with multiple subspecialty teams. Each of these teams is composed of residents, advance practice providers, and attendings.

RESULTS (THEMES)

This study probed into the heart of a critical moment in direct-care nursing and shares the story behind barriers to code reduction and the cultural influences that have an impact on clinical decision making in escalating situations. Nurse participants identified some common facilitators and barriers to calling RRTs or intervening before a code event during their interviews; these are outlined in **Table 2**.

Because many RRT calls do not lead to the patient being transferred to an ICU, staff may begin to view that RRT call as unnecessary or even as a failure and be less likely to

	Theme
Table 2	
Common facilitators and barriers	
Facilitators	Availability of experienced nurse resources for consultation
	• "[The nurse is] still worried and will probably go to the charge nurse."
	Nurses have good clinical recognition skills
	• "I trust my colleagues to recognize things."
	Strong culture of nurse assertion
	• "Whenever I don't feel good about something or I'm concerned about a patient, I'll communicate it with everybody and I'll do whatever I need to make that patient better."
	Supportive nursing leadership and RRT responders
	• "I really do believe our unit is a very supportive unit, and I think our charge nurses are excellent. I mean when I became a charge nurse I modeled myself right after them because I think they do a great job in supporting us, I really do."
Barriers	Capacity/bed availability in the ICU
	• "The nurses have a sick kid,...but they're like "well, the PICU's full they won't take him anyways, and I think that's a huge barrier"."
	Equipment issues
	• "Portable monitor wasn't working."
	• "We don't have cardorespiratory (CR) monitors in every room."
	Newer, less experienced, nurses and doctors/residents may be less likely to initiate an RRT or code blue without consulting someone more experienced.
	• "As a new grad you didn't want to be wrong because you felt that was a failure if you were wrong."
	• "You go to newer residents and if they have to send a patient downstairs [to the ICU] it's like they have done something wrong. They feel like they missed something, they didn't do a good treatment plan."
	Physician and nurse dynamics (ie, previous bad experiences with communication or escalation, knowing the provider vs working with someone for the first time)
	• "It's easier to tell the senior [resident] that we've had the relationship with for the 2 or 3 y, I'm still worried I'm gonna call the RRT."
	Mistrust of objective clinical triggers, abnormal vital signs, or assessment findings became the new baseline for patients instead of them continuing to be triggers for escalating care
	• "Well this is what this patient has been doing."
	• "They just go up and down...it's part of the course."
	Acuity level of patients, feels like a step-down unit
	• "There are times that I feel like we are the step down unit, that we have kids that you're like this kid really should be in ICU."

call in a similar situation in the future. There was a strong cultural phenomenon of the staff and medical teams wanting to try all the interventions they could for their patients prior to calling an RRT to see if the patients would improve. In addition, there are expectations to escalate concerns up the chain of command, which was identified as a barrier. This clinical chain of escalation may delay the process of activating an RRT or code blue.

The research team found one theme in the interview transcripts to be especially intriguing. Nurses described that they had a strong culture of assertion and felt comfortable escalating their concerns about a patient. On review of the interview transcripts, however, the researchers identified several situations that nurses described as exemplifying strong assertion yet revealed behaviors that unit leaders on the research team regard as inadequate assertion. In the interview stories, the nurses tended to fall short of escalating their concerns to the highest levels necessary in situations when the nurses' opinion was in conflict with the resident/provider opinion about whether to call an RRT or not.

When concerned for clinical deterioration, all 10 nurse participants described that the first step was to page the medical team starting with the lowest-ranking resident. If the resident did not concur that an RRT call was warranted, in most instances the nurse's next step was to work toward convincing for agreement. **Fig. 1** provides a visual depiction of how nurses may get caught up in a cycle of attempting to convince the provider to agree with them that an RRT is necessary or to continue to communicate their concerns until they feel validated and affirmed to take the next step of

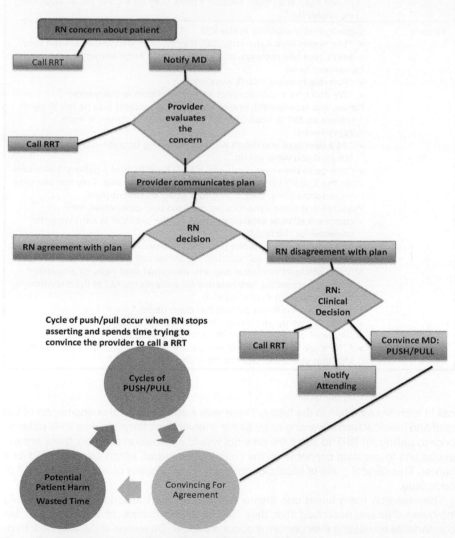

Fig. 1. Escalation communication patterns of registered nurses.

activation of RRT. This hesitation to activate an RRT until the team is on board causes delays in escalating care and, in addition, diverts the nurse's attention away from other assigned patients.

The following example from the interview transcripts exemplifies several barriers to nursing activation of rapid response, including the dangerous waste of time that occurs in the cycle of push-pull, illustrated in **Fig. 1**. This interview participant describes an incident when serving as charge nurse. She says:

...one of my nurses came to me concerned about the increased work of breathing on a little 18 month old. And that his heart rate was up, and his respirs [respiration rate was] up but he was starting to retract, and she just felt like he wasn't doing very good. He went up about a liter and a half of oxygen in an hour. He just wasn't looking right.

The patient's nurse relayed to the charge nurse that she had "tried to talk" to the first-year resident, who stated he would see the 18-month old after completing rounds. The nurse was "frustrated," certain that the child needed an RRT evaluation or to transfer to the ICU. The charge nurse intervenes by calling the first-year resident herself and received the same response. The charge nurse asserts by going up the chain of command:

...I called the senior, and I said, "Look, you know, I have looked at this baby and ...we want to call an RRT but we're getting a lot of pushback from the first year."

The charge nurse goes on to tell the interviewer "...when we override the doctors, that's a big issue around here. You know, that's just something you don't want to do, you really want to have that teamwork piece." The interviewee continues:

...The senior said he would send the first year up. So, we waited about a half an hour. Nothing was happening. ...And then I called the attending. You know, I said, "Look we're really having an issue, we need somebody to come up and look at this kid."

The attending physician directed the first-year resident to the see the patient. The interviewee estimates that about 2 hours passed from the time of the first call placed by the nurse until this physician saw the patient. The charge nurse observed the resident's interaction with the patient's nurse. She recalls:

And this is really subjective, but he seemed to have a lot of attitude. It was, you know, "You didn't have to call my attending." I said, "Well, you know what? We weren't getting a response from you or the senior, the senior said he'd send you up, and you didn't come. ...[M]y nurse has ...a concern and I need you to respond to that." So [the patient's nurse] started talking and he kept interrupting her, and I had to step in and say... "I really wish you'd just let her finish talking so she can tell you what her concerns are." He kind of rolled his eyes and looked at me, and I said, "Um, so should I just call the senior? ...[I]f you're not going to listen to her then this is kind of a waste of time, and communication is breaking down, and she's frustrated, and you're frustrated, so should I just call somebody else." He said, "No, I will listen." So he did. And he assessed the patient. He didn't feel like the patient needed an RRT, but she still did, so we called it. And they ended up taking the kiddo downstairs [to the pediatric ICU (PICU) where]...he was put on CPAP [continuous positive airway pressure] pretty fast.

This story ends well for the patient but only after the nurse and charge nurse tolerate considerable risk during the 2-hour wait to provide an opportunity for a physician to assess the child prior to initiating an RRT. Other participants described similar stories and offered the following statements:

- "I think it's a collaboration but I think the nurses, we just have a hard time calling it [RRT] without them [providers] supporting that decision."
- "It doesn't feel good to have the doctor kind of be upset with you or angry with you."
- "I didn't feel supported by the resident."
- [Resident's actions are] "saying your assessment is not valid to me."

Nurses might make a second call to a resident and/or senior resident when concerned about their patient but many of the stories lacked escalation to a fellow or attending provider.

- "...even some senior residents... are offended if you want to go up the chain of command and that you have to assert. I think they feel like it's a failure on their part."

Participants described first-year residents as the most difficult to convince and having the most hierarchical attitudes. Nurses observed first-year residents who displayed negative attitudes and resistance to take nurses' concerns seriously. Attending physicians and midlevel providers who lead the unit's medical teams were reported to be highly considerate of nursing, even to the point of offering to call the RRT for the sole purpose of alleviating the nurses' concerns by bringing in "a second set of eyes."

DISCUSSION

Close examination of nurses' past experiences with early clinical intervention efforts helped reveal facilitators and barriers to code reduction. This research has provided insight for the development of future quality improvement interventions to reduce codes on these units and increase patient safety.

Nurses spend the most time with patients who are hospitalized. Their voice for prevention measures to code reduction are integral to the success of quality improvement efforts. This study identified many facilitators to code reduction, including availability of experienced registered nurse (RN) resources, nurses having good clinical recognition skills, strong culture of assertion, and supportive nursing leadership and RRT teams. Diving into the heart of nursing allowed this research to identify some important barriers to code reduction. This study revealed similar themes to what other publications reported, such as capacity/bed availability, equipment issues, treating the inpatient unit as a step-down unit, mistrust of clinical triggers, and physician/nursing dynamics.[5,7-9] Shearer and colleagues[7] found that a rapid response call was not activated in 42% of instances despite clinical triggers. Sociocultural factors, such as intraprofessional hierarchy, also has an impact on why staff do not activate RRTs.[7]

Triangulation occurred when the themes from this study and Reese and colleagues[9] study were compared and validated with interdisciplinary teams throughout the hospital. The themes were validated using focus group methodology. These focus groups consisted of nurses, physicians from both PICU and medical units (representing all levels—residents, fellows, advanced practice providers, and attendings), respiratory therapists, and pharmacists. Discussion of the research themes allowed for the researchers and code committee to identify appropriate interventions to impact code reduction throughout the organization.

LIMITATIONS

Four limitations were identified in this study. First, 2 members of the study team were known to the participants. Although effort was made to protect the confidentiality of participants, this could have had an impact on their willingness to speak up and fully reflect their perceptions of code reduction measures. Second, no new-graduate RNs volunteered to participate. Several participants started their nursing career on the unit as new-graduate nurses. Next, all the participants perceived themselves as assertive nurses causing the research team to wonder if they may not have captured the voice of the nonassertive nurse. Lastly, this study took place on the medical unit in a pediatric hospital and may not be generalizable to other areas.

SUMMARY

Code reduction efforts and the addition of RRTs have improved patient outcomes in hospitals. This study describes some cultural impacts that can potentially impede code reduction and utilization of RRTs. Nurses often assert but are faced with barriers when they have to assert up the clinical chain of command. These barriers can have an impact on their willingness to continue to assert when they have to maneuver through the hierarchical system found within hospitals. Furthermore, nurses waste time attempting to convince providers to agree with their concerns about a patient before activating an RRT. In situations where code rates are stagnant or not declining, a hospital should consider looking deeper into the cultural aspects on the unit to determine where potential barriers exist. This study shows interventions beyond RRT and team training may be needed to have an impact on code reduction within hospitals. Analyzing the barriers and facilitators to code reduction can assist in identifying appropriate interventions within a particular unit.

ACKNOWLEDGMENTS

Co-investigator: Anne Marie Kotzer, PhD, FAAN, RN; Code Committee Chair: Beth Wathen, MS, PNP, CCRN; Registered Nurses on the Inpatient Medical Unit at Children's Hospital Colorado; Division of Nursing Leadership: Brenda Hyle, BSN, RN; and Traci Link, MS, RN.

REFERENCES

1. Hillman K, Chen J, Cretikos M, et al. Introduction of the medical emergency team (MET) system: a cluster-randomised controlled trial. Lancet 2005;365(9477): 2091–7.
2. Johnston MJ, Arora S, King D, et al. A systematic review to identify the factors that affect failure to rescue and escalation of care in surgery. Surgery 2015;157(4): 752–63.
3. Cioffi J, Conwayt R, Everist L, et al. 'Patients of concern' to nurses in acute care settings: a descriptive study. Aust Crit Care 2009;22(4):178–86.
4. Minick P, Harvey S. The early recognition of patient problems among medical-surgical nurses. Medsurg Nurs 2003;12(5):291–7.
5. Cioffi J. Nurses' experiences of making decisions to call emergency assistance to their patients. J Adv Nurs 2000;32(1):108–14.
6. Braaten JS. CE: Original research: hospital system barriers to rapid response team activation: a cognitive work analysis. Am J Nurs 2015;115(2):22–32.
7. Shearer B, Marshall S, Buist MD, et al. What stops hospital clinical staff from following protocols? An analysis of the incidence and factors behind the failure

of bedside clinical staff to activate the rapid response system in a multi-campus Australian metropolitan healthcare service. BMJ Qual Saf 2012;21(7):569–75.

8. Roberts KE, Bonafide CP, Paine CW, et al. Barriers to calling for urgent assistance despite a comprehensive pediatric rapid response system. Am J Crit Care 2014; 23(3):223–9.

9. Reese J, Simmons R, Barnard J. Assertion practices and beliefs among nurses and physicians on an inpatient pediatric medical unit. Hosp Pediatr 2016;6(5): 275–81.

10. Prado R, Albert RK, Mehler PS, et al. Rapid response: a quality improvement conundrum. J Hosp Med 2009;4(4):255–7.

11. Tait D. Nursing recognition and response to signs of clinical deterioration. Nurs Manag (Harrow) 2010;17(6):31–5.

12. Andrews T, Waterman H. Packaging: a grounded theory of how to report physiological deterioration effectively. J Adv Nurs 2005;52(5):473–81.

13. Robb G, Seddon M. A multi-faceted approach to the physiologically unstable patient. Qual Saf Health Care 2010;19(5):e47.

Case Study of High-Dose Ketamine for Treatment of Complex Regional Pain Syndrome in the Pediatric Intensive Care Unit

CrossMark

Tracy Ann Pasek, RN, MSN, DNP, CCNS, CCRN, CIMI[a],*,
Kelli Crowley, PharmD, BCPS, BCPPS[b], Catherine Campese, RN, MSN, CPNP[c],
Rachel Lauer, RN, MSN, FNP-BC[c], Charles Yang, MD[c]

KEYWORDS

- Complex regional pain syndrome • Pediatric • Pain • Ketamine
- Pediatric critical care • Pediatric intensive care unit
- Pharmacologic pain management • Advanced practice nursing

KEY POINTS

- Refractory pediatric CRPS is not a common development but when it occurs, there are significant physical, psychological and social effects.
- Interest has expanded to include ketamine's potential role in the treatment of chronic pain syndromes such as complex regional pain syndrome.
- Preparing for the admission of a patient with CRPS to the PICU for pain management presented a unique opportunity for collaboration among advanced practice nurses.

INTRODUCTION

Complex regional pain syndrome (CRPS) is a life-altering and debilitating chronic pain condition. A hallmark symptom of CRPS is severe neuropathic pain that is disproportionate to pain that would be expected of an associated or causal injury.[1] In fact, a patient may not recall experiencing an injury to an extremity, for example, that involved soft tissue or peripheral nerves before being diagnosed with CRPS.[1]

[a] Pain, Pediatric Intensive Care Unit, Evidence-Based Practice and Research, Children's Hospital of Pittsburgh, University of Pittsburgh Medical Center, Pittsburgh, PA, USA; [b] Department of Pharmacy, Children's Hospital of Pittsburgh, University of Pittsburgh Medical Center, Pittsburgh, PA, USA; [c] Department of Anesthesiology, Children's Hospital of Pittsburgh, University of Pittsburgh Medical Center, Pittsburgh, PA, USA
* Corresponding author. PICU-Critical Care Nursing Administration, Children's Hospital of Pittsburgh, University of Pittsburgh Medical Center, 4401 Penn Avenue, Pittsburgh, PA 15224.
E-mail address: Tracy.Pasek@chp.edu

Crit Care Nurs Clin N Am 29 (2017) 177–186
http://dx.doi.org/10.1016/j.cnc.2017.01.005
0899-5885/17/© 2017 Elsevier Inc. All rights reserved.
ccnursing.theclinics.com

Characteristics of pain associated with CRPS include allodynia or pain evoked from what would ordinarily be nonpainful stimuli.[1] More specifically, mecanoallodynia is pain from light touch or pressure to a body part (eg, a pat on the arm).[1] Changes in skin temperature can also result in pain known as thermal allodynia.[1] Hyperalgesia or extreme sensitivity to pain is also part of CRPS. Additionally, a patient may experience hyperpathia. Hyperpathia occurs when repeated or prolonged nonpainful stimuli become perceived as painful.[1]

We present a case study of a female who received high-dose ketamine for the management of her CRPS. The innovative treatment lies not only within the pharmacologic management of her pain, but in the fact that she was the first patient to be admitted to our pediatric intensive care unit (PICU) solely for pain control. Furthermore, she was a young adult and not a pediatric patient (>21 years of age). The coordination of her pre-admission care required remarkable planning. The patient's positive outcomes at discharge from the hospital to a rehabilitation setting were compelling. Although we comprehensively addressed the "four pillars of CRPS treatment," this paper has as its foci the pillars of pain relief and the support of the patient's self-management.[2,3]

METHODS

We provided direct care to this patient. Additionally, we conducted a retrospective chart review.

CASE

The patient was treated with a high-dose intravenous ketamine infusion and 2 lumbar epidural catheters during her 22-day PICU stay. Her pain intensity at its worst was reported as 7 out of 10 using a self-report pain assessment scale. Ketamine was slowly titrated from 10 mg/h to 110 mg/h over a period of 11 days. After the fourth day of ketamine therapy and after the placement of epidural catheters infusing ropivacaine 0.1%, she experienced decreased pain. Moreover, she was able to tolerate having her left lower extremity touched. Initially, we used lidocaine 2% in the epidurals, but this was not tolerated. Changing to ropivacaine 0.1% was a key turning point for the patient and her pain remained stable with the lowest intensity of 5 out of 10.

Initial progress was evidenced by her ability to roll side to side with minimal assistance. The patient reported relief of hand dystonia. She experienced ketamine-related adverse effects, including decreased appetite and a mild sensation of bladder fullness, despite a urinary catheter during epidural therapy. She experienced dysphoria and hallucinations with the lidocaine 2% therapy until it was discontinued. The patient reported having vivid dreams and she became somnolent when her ketamine dose was titrated to doses near 100 mg/h. We used midazolam to combat the adverse side effects of ketamine and this was effective. Overall, the patient tolerated the intravenous ketamine infusion well with aggressive control of adverse effects.

We initiated physical therapy on day 1 of her PICU stay. Once her pain decreased, she began tolerating the physical therapy with fewer complaints. She had good strength and motion of all extremities because the epidurals enhanced the outcomes of physical therapy. She became very motivated to progress with the vigilant support of her family. By the second week of hospitalization, she was sitting upright in a cardiac chair for hours at a time. She did not experience syncopal events in the cardiac chair or with other physical therapy interventions.

The epidural therapy was weaned after 9 days and she did not experience pain escalation with this. After removal of the epidural catheters, the ketamine infusion was continued another for another day, at which time the patient was weaned to an oral formulation. She tolerated this well. Once weaned, we facilitated her transfer to a local specialized rehabilitation center for continued general rehabilitation before returning to her home. The patient's goals for rehabilitation are listed in **Box 1**. Her family assisted her with writing these because she was unable to hold a writing implement. We recommend including a patient's goals in the medical record because they represent milestones the patient wants to achieve rather than providers' goals for the patient. A comparison of the patient's progress is summarized in **Table 1**.

One symptom that was never resolved for the patient was photosensitivity. This was present on admission to the PICU and persisted throughout her hospital course and discharge. She preferred wearing sunglasses for self-management of photosensitivity. The patient's duration of stay totaled 22 days.

THE BUDAPEST CLINICAL DIAGNOSIS FOR CHRONIC REGIONAL PAIN SYNDROME

Our chronic pain service uses the Budapest Criteria to guide the clinical diagnosis for CRPS. The Budapest criteria include 4 major points: (A) a patient experiences continual pain that is disproportionate to the provoking event, (B) a patient has at least 1 sign in 2 or more categories (sensory, vasomotor, sudomotor/edema, motor/trophic), (C) a patient complains of at least 1 symptom in 3 of the aforementioned categories, and (D) a patient's signs and symptoms cannot be explained by a diagnosis other than CRPS.[3,4]

According to these criteria, the sensory category includes allodynia and/or hyperalgesia.[3,4] The vasomotor category is manifest by temperature asymmetry and/or color changes and/or color asymmetry.[3,4] Sudomotor/edema is the third category and includes edema and/or changes in sweating and/or asymmetrical sweating.[3,4] Last, motor/trophic changes or dysfunction comprise the fourth category.[3,4] A patient may experience decreased range of motion, weakness, tremor, dystonia, and trophic changes to nails, skin, and hair.[3,4]

INTRAVENOUS KETAMINE DOSING PROCEDURE

A dosing procedure that was developed by the hospital's chronic pain service and approved by the pharmacy and therapeutics committee guided therapy for this patient. The main components of the guideline include (1) the purpose of ketamine, (2) the definition of ketamine, (3) general guidelines, (4) equipment for the administration of ketamine, (5) the procedure for the administration of ketamine, and (6) requirements for the assessment and documentation of pain intensity and sedation level. The management of adverse events is also part of the dosing procedure and these include

---

Box 1
Patient's goals for rehabilitation

- Accomplish self-care independently (eg, bathe, dress, shampoo hair, wash hands at sink)
- Transition from bed pan to bedside toilet
- Go outdoors for activities other than medical appointments
- Learn how to operate a powered wheelchair
- Transfer to and from a powered wheelchair
- Experience reduced photosensitivity

Table 1 Progress with activities of daily living after ketamine therapy	
Before Hospitalization	**At Discharge from Hospital to Rehabilitation Unit**
Total restriction to bed for ≥3 y	Transferring to and from cardiac chair independently; assistance required to protect intravenous tubing connections only
Hands in a fist position from dystonia	Hands almost fully open and extended
Unable to give/receive hugs owing to severe pain and syncope	Able to give/receive hugs without severe pain and syncope
Needed assistance with position changes in bed	Independently changes position in bed using the side rails for support
Limited endurance for activity	Improved endurance for activity; able to sit in cardiac chair for a minimum of 3 h
Arms propped with pillows to eat, brush teeth owing to limited shoulder function	Improved shoulder function; able to lift arms to eat, brush teeth; propping with pillows unnecessary

hallucinations, dysphoria, agitation, hypertension, oversedation, urinary retention, and nausea and vomiting.

The general guideline portion of the dosing procedure begins with education and preparation of the child and family. Dose and pump verification is outlined specifically for patient safety purposes. The location wherein high-dose ketamine therapy may be administered is described (eg, nonintensive care units) as well as monitoring recommendations. Doses for the initiation of the ketamine infusion, subsequent infusion, duration of infusion, and recovery are listed along with assessment parameters and a process for notifying key personnel if a patient problem occurs. Anticipatory guidance regarding the clinical indication for ketamine is delineated. For example, "Patients with complex regional pain syndrome may require 5 days of ketamine infusion therapy."

PHARMACOLOGIC MANAGEMENT

The primary component of the pharmacotherapy treatment strategy plan was the escalating dose ketamine infusion via patient-controlled analgesia. Adjunctive drug therapies such as local anesthetic epidurals and benzodiazepines were used as needed (**Table 2**). Additionally, all preintervention maintenance medications were continued throughout admission as prescribed before admission (**Box 2**).

Upon admission, the patient was started on ketamine 10 mg/mL intravenously with an initial continuous infusion rate of 10 mg/h and was permitted 10 mg demand doses every 15 minutes as needed. On day 2, the patient received fourteen 10-mg demand

Table 2 Adjunct medication therapy	
Epidural lidocaine	Days 6–9
Epidural ropivacaine	Days 9–15
Diazepam 6 mg IV every 4 h	Days 1–2
Diazepam 10 mg IV every 4 h	Day 3
Diazepam 10 mg PO every 6 h	Days 16–18
Midazolam 2 mg IV every 2 h	Days 3–16

> **Box 2**
> **Maintenance medications prescribed throughout hospitalization**
>
> - Baclofen 20 mg PO 4 times a day
> - Dantrolene 25 mg PO daily
> - Duloxetine 60 mg PO daily
> - Melatonin 15 mg PO daily at bedtime
> - Pregabalin 75 mg PO 2 times a day
> - Tizanidine 10 mg PO daily at bedtime
> - Naltrexone 7.5 mg PO daily
> - Clonidine 0.1 mg PO 2 times a day
> - Diphenhydramine 50 mg PO 4 times a day as needed (until 2/19/2016)
> - Diphenhydramine 50 mg PO 4 times a day (beginning 2/19/2016)
> - Naproxen 250 mg PO 2 times a day as needed

doses and on day 3 the demand dose was increased to 20 mg per dose. A rapid dosing escalation of between 5 and 20 mg/h per day occurred daily over the next 10 days (**Fig. 1**). Dose adjustments were determined each day based on patient tolerability. Some sedation, lethargy, and confusion were experienced through days 7, 8, and 9, necessitating smaller incremental increases. The patient did continue to request demand doses and received an average of 9 doses per day over the first 9 days. A maximum infusion rate of 110 mg/h was achieved on day 10 and continued for approximately 3.5 days. During the 24-hour periods of days 11, 12, and 13, the patient received a total of 2640 mg of ketamine as continuous infusion and a cumulative amount of 2700 mg each day when demand doses were accounted for. This was followed by a rapid wean over the next 72 hours, at which point she was transitioned to oral ketamine maintenance therapy of 50 mg 4 times a day. It took 17 days to complete this treatment. Further weaning was planned to occur over an extended period of time on an outpatient basis.

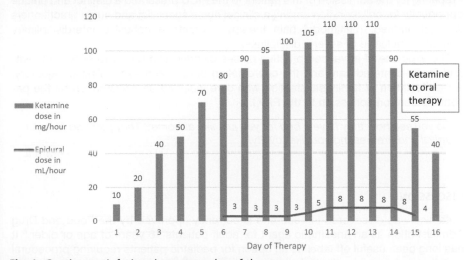

Fig. 1. Continuous infusion dose versus day of therapy.

On day 6, it was determined that the ketamine therapy would be supplemented with local anesthetic epidural therapy, so catheters were placed at the L1-L2 and L3-L4 positions (see **Fig. 1**). Lidocaine 2% preservative-free parenteral solution was the first agent used. Each catheter was initiated at 3 mL/h continuous infusion with additional 4-mL demand doses available hourly. The patient received 17, 23, and 15 demand doses in both catheters on days 6, 7, and 8, respectively. Day 9, a serum lidocaine level was drawn to assess the degree of systemic absorption. The result was 4.3 µg/mL. A range of 1.5 to 5.0 µg/mL is considered therapeutic when lidocaine is administered as an antiarrhythmic agent. Systemic absorption is undesirable when lidocaine is used for local effect, so to avoid adverse effects or cardiac toxicity, the epidural medication was switched to ropivacaine 0.1% preservative-free parenteral solution. The initial orders were for 3 mL/h through 1 catheter and 4 mL/h through the other with the option of 3 mL-doses on demand each hour as needed. Continuous epidural rates were rapidly escalated to 8 mL/h at each site and demand doses of 4 mL. This escalation took place on day 10 and remained until day 14. Frequent demand doses were administered on days 9 through 12 with a maximum of 24 doses on day 10. The continuous rate was decreased by 50% on day 15 and discontinued on the following day.

Benzodiazepines were used as adjunct therapy to control adverse effects of dysphoria or anxiety. Diazepam was ordered at 6 mg IV every 6 hours around the clock but the dosing interval was shortened to every 4 hours by the evening of the first day of ketamine treatment. The dose was increased to 10 mg on the same schedule by day 3. At this point it was decided to try switching to midazolam at 2 mg IV every 2 hours as needed to see if efficacy improved. The patient received 4 doses within the first 24 hours then decreased to 1 to 2 doses per day after that. As the rate of the ketamine infusion neared the maximum dosage, the number of midazolam doses per day increased with 7 doses administered on day 11, 5 doses on days 12 and 13 each, and 4 doses given on day 14. Once the ketamine infusion was discontinued on day 16, midazolam was discontinued and diazepam reordered, 10 mg PO every 6 hours as needed. There were no oral diazepam doses documented throughout the remainder of the admission.

ADVANCED PRACTICE NURSE COLLABORATION

Preparing for the admission of this patient to the PICU presented a distinct and unique opportunity for collaboration among a clinical nurse specialist and nurse practitioners (**Box 3**). Indeed, multimodal pain therapy warrants a cohesive interdisciplinary approach, inclusive of several disciplines.

The expertise of advanced practice nurses blended exquisitely to ensure patient- and family-centered care and the coordination of care across the illness trajectory. A manifestation of family satisfaction with care included an exclamation by the patient's parent on admission to the PICU.

Do you see how they have a bed for you just like at home? They planned for your arrival and are treating you like royalty!

—Parent

DISCUSSION

Ketamine was discovered in 1962 and is currently approved by the Food and Drug Administration as an anesthetic agent for adult patients 16 years of age or older.[5] It has long been useful off label as an option for pediatric patients requiring procedural sedation and as an anesthetic in the operating room.[6–9] More recently, it has served in

---

Box 3
Planning by advanced practice nurses for the admission of a patient with complex regional pain syndrome to the pediatric intensive care unit

1. Collaborate with the pain service, critical care medicine service, physical therapy, PICU leadership, and third-party payers.

2. Develop trust with the patient and family.

3. Coordinate transport (eg, prehospital providers, an organization's transport team).

4. Use the unique expertise of unit-based pharmacists regarding dosing (eg, ketamine, local anesthetic) and adherence to an established guideline.

5. Prepare and lead interdisciplinary education about chronic regional pain syndrome.

6. Anticipate and address concerns regarding pain culture (eg, provide resources to a unit manager to support staff nurses' provision of compassionate care).

7. Conduct an assessment of needs and routines at home to facilitate normalcy in the (eg, specialty support surface).

8. Assess the patient's and family's goals for the PICU admission and document them in the medical record.

9. Assess the patient's primary care concerns (eg, excruciating pain with light touch; extreme light sensitivity without sun glasses) and communicate them to providers.

Abbreviation: PICU, pediatric intensive care unit.

---

the PICU to provide or augment sedation and analgesia management, particularly in mechanically ventilated patients.[10,11] Interest has expanded to include ketamine's potential role in the treatment of chronic pain syndromes such as traumatic peripheral nerve injury, postherpetic pain, spinal cord injury, a variety of neuropathic pains, and CRPS.[12]

The mechanism of ketamine is inhibition of N-methyl-D-aspartate (NMDA) and other receptors, including opioid. Ketamine is highly lipophilic and crosses the blood–brain barrier rapidly after administration allowing for direct action on the cortex and limbic system and quick onset of effect.[12] Metabolism occurs in the liver through the cytochrome P450 system producing metabolites, norketamine and 4-, 5- and 6-hydroxynorketamine. It is not known if these metabolites play a part in long-term analgesic effects.[12] It seems that the duration of infusion is in direct relation to the duration of effect observed in CRPS patients.[13]

An optimal recommendation for ketamine dosing for CRPS therapy has been elusive. Literature pertaining to the adult population is limited; for children, it is nonexistent. In adults, an array of dosing strategies has produced variable degrees of efficacy, rates of remission, sustainability, and return of function. Currently there are 2 approaches to ketamine dosing: subanesthetic versus anesthetic. Sigtermans and colleagues[13] treated 30 adults with an average disease duration of 7.4 years with a 4-day, low-dose ketamine infusion (subanesthetic) initiated at 1.2 μg/kg/min and titrated to a maximum of 7.2 μg/kg/min. Patients were found to have significant pain relief for approximately 12 weeks but no functional improvement. Correll and colleagues[14] conducted a retrospective study of 33 subjects and revealed a 75% rate of complete pain relief with 2 patients with no effect. Remission lasted for at least 3 months for 54% of patients and at least 6 months for another 31% of patients. Dosing was subanesthetic between 10 and 25 mg/h in 78% of infusion treatments with 5 poor responders escalating to a maximum of 50 mg/h for over a period of 2 to 5 days on average.[14] There were no clinically significant adverse effects described in these 2 publications.[13,14] Conversely, Kiefer and colleagues[15] evaluated subanesthetic ketamine dosing titrated from 50 mg/d up to 500 mg/d in 4 refractory patients with no pain relief or improvement in symptoms. Anesthetic dosing of 3 to 7 mg/kg/h of ketamine for 5 days was successful for significant reduction of pain in all patients in trials by Kiefer and colleagues[16] and Koffler and colleagues.[1] Kiefer's team[16] reported 100% of 20 patients were in complete remission at 1 month and 80% remained in remission after 6 months. Many patients in Kiefer's cohort also reported improved quality of life, movement, and ability to work, which is in stark contrast with Koffler's subjects.[1,16]

Ketamine therapy is not without drawbacks; there is a lengthy side effect profile associated with this drug. Toxicities associated with ketamine use primarily affect the central nervous, hepatic, and cardiovascular systems.[5] Hallucinations, anxiety, paranoia, intense dreams, and nightmares are experienced commonly by patients and can be quite profound. Drowsiness, dizziness, and sedation can occur 20% to 25% of the time.[17] Patients require frequent evaluation of mental status. Benzodiazepines, often midazolam and clonidine, may be used to temper these psychological effects, but they will not eliminate them.[12] Additionally, ketamine is known to stimulate the sympathetic system resulting in hypertension and an elevated heart rate. Patients should undergo continuous electrocardiogram and blood pressure monitoring throughout duration of therapy when receiving high-doses continuously, necessitating intensive care–level nursing care. There is no generally accepted drug therapy to counter this activation of the cardiovascular system, although clonidine may be helpful.[12] Hepatotoxicity is the other primary concern when ketamine is administered for prolonged periods or repeatedly. Noppers and colleagues[18] had to abandon their exploratory trial investigating the use of ketamine therapy in CRPS-1 patients owing to the development of hepatitis in 3 (50%) of the first 6 patients enrolled. Despite this finding there are few other case reports of hepatotoxicity in the literature. Although the guidelines do not provide recommendations, monitoring of liver enzyme levels should occur. Additionally, it is not known what the long-term effects of repeated ketamine therapy will be or if it might be dose dependent. Last but not least, it must be noted that ketamine dependence can develop and is a known drug of abuse.

Ketamine, especially in higher doses, is known to depress respiratory drive. Although there is no one standard dosing strategy for CRPS therapy, all patients undergoing these regimens receive quantities of medication that exceed routine sedation and analgesia dosing. Care must be used in nonintubated and nonmechanically ventilated patients owing to risks of cardiopulmonary compromise. Monitoring includes continuous transcutaneous oxygen saturation. Treatment should occur only in environments where experienced personnel are readily available for urgent situations requiring supportive ventilation.[5] Patients prescribed lower dosing regimens may be able to receive each dose or treatment in a hospital outpatient clinic or as an inpatient on an acute care unit if resuscitative equipment is present; however, high-dose regimens (eg, anesthetic dosing) should be done in the PICU. Because the case patient's dose was to be titrated to the highest rate tolerated, it was decided that the safest location for our patient would be the PICU. It was not anticipated that intubation necessary during this admission, and it was not.

When developing an intravenous ketamine dosing procedure, we recommend cross-referencing all relevant patient care policies for consistency. These policies may include the patient-controlled analgesia policy owing to the pump and tubing that are used. The pain assessment, sedation assessment, and medication administration policies should be cross-referenced for patient safety. Last, patient care policies pertaining to documentation should align with the ketamine dosing procedure for patient safety and regulatory purposes.

SUMMARY

Refractory pediatric CRPS is not a common development, but when it occurs, there are significant physical, psychological, and social effects. Continuous infusion ketamine is reserved for patients who fail more conventional treatment options owing to risks related to adverse effects and the need for hospital admission. The therapy can be very effective at inducing long-term remission; however, it is associated with complexities including intensive nursing care requirements and toxicity monitoring to insure comfort and safety in these oft debilitated patients.

The successful outcomes for the patient at discharge from the hospital to a rehabilitation unit are compared in **Table 1**. It is noteworthy that emotional progress was measured. Certainly, independent personal hygiene is basic and important, yet giving and receiving hugs was of particular significance for this young woman and her family. Perhaps one of the most poignant images of this patient's emotional progress during hospitalization was a photograph taken at discharge wherein she was smiling and giving a "thumbs up" as she was surrounded by pet therapy animals . . . that she was hugging.

REFERENCES

1. Koffler SP, Hampstead BM, Irani F, et al. The neurocognitive effects of 5 day anesthetic ketamine for the treatment of refractory complex regional pain syndrome. Arch Clin Neuropsychol 2007;22:719–29.
2. Turner-Stokes L, Goebel A. Complex regional pain syndrome in adults: concise guidance. (On behalf of the Guideline Development Group of the Royal College of Physicians). Clin Med 2011;11:596–600.
3. Ganty P, Chawla R. Complex regional pain syndrome: recent updates. Contin Educ Anaesth Crit Care Pain 2014;14(2):79–84.
4. Goebel A. CRPS in adults. Rheumatology 2011;50:1739–50.
5. Ketamine hydrochloride injection, solution [package insert]. Rockford, IL: Mylan Institutional LLC; 2012.
6. Schwartz KR, Fredricks K, Al Tawil Z, et al. An innovative safe anesthesia and analgesia package for emergency pediatric procedures and surgeries when no anesthetist is available. Int J Emerg Med 2016;9(1):16.
7. Kannikeswaran N, Lieh-Lai M, Malian M, et al. Optimal dosing of intravenous ketamine for procedural sedation in children in the ED – a randomized controlled trial. Am J Emerg Med 2016;34(8):1347–53.
8. Cote CJ, Lerman J, Anderson B, editors. A practice of anesthesia for infants and children. 5th edition. Philadelphia: Elsevier Saunders; 2013.
9. Lin C, Durieux ME. Ketamine and kids: an update. Paediatr Anaesth 2005;15(2): 91–7.
10. Tobias JD. Sedation and analgesia in paediatric intensive care units: a guide to drug selection and use. Paediatr Drugs 1999;1(2):109–26.
11. Lowrie L, Weiss AH, Lacombe C. The pediatric sedation unit: a mechanism for pediatric sedation. Pediatrics 1998;102(3):E30.
12. Neisters M, Martini C, Dahan A. Ketamine for chronic pain: risks and benefits. Br J Clin Pharmacol 2013;77(2):357–67.

13. Sigtermans MJ, van Hilten JJ, Bauer MC, et al. Ketamine produces effective and long-term pain relief in patients with complex regional pain syndrome type 1. Pain 2009;145:304–11.

14. Correll GE, Maleki J, Gracely EJ, et al. Subanesthetic ketamine infusion therapy: a retrospective analysis of a novel therapeutic approach to complex regional pain syndrome. Pain Med 2004;5(3):263–75.

15. Kiefer RT, Rohr P, Ploppa A, et al. A pilot open-label study of the efficacy of subanesthetic isomeric s(+) ketamine in refractory CRPS patients. Pain Med 2008; 9(1):44–54.

16. Kiefer RT, Rohr P, Ploppa A, et al. Efficacy of ketamine in anesthetic dosage for the treatment of refractory complex regional pain syndrome: an open-label phase II Study. Pain Med 2008;9(8):1173–201.

17. Cvrcek P. Side effects of ketamine in the long-term treatment of neuropathic pain. Pain Med 2008;9:253–7.

18. Noppers I, Niesters M, Aarts L, et al. Ketamine for the treatment of chronic non-cancer pain. Expert Opin Pharmacother 2010;11(4):2417–29.

Airways and Injuries

Protecting Our Pediatric Patients from Respiratory Device-Related Pressure Injuries

Laura J. Miske, RN, MSN, CNS[a],*, Molly Stetzer, RN, BSN, CWOCN[b],
Melissa Garcia, RN, MSN, ACCNS-P[c],
Judith J. Stellar, RN, MSN, CRNP, PPCNP-BC, CWOCN[d]

KEYWORDS

- Tracheostomy ties • Tracheostomy securement devices
- Noninvasive ventilation (NIPPV) • Pressure ulcer medical device
- Hospital-acquired pressure injury (HAPI) • Pressure injury prevention
- Incidence tracking

KEY POINTS

- Pressure injury prevention is imperative in contemporary value-based health care.
- Device-related pressure injuries are the majority of pressure injuries in pediatric hospitals.
- Respiratory device–related pressure injuries are especially challenging given the life-sustaining nature of the therapy.

INTRODUCTION

Noninvasive positive pressure ventilation (NIPPV) and tracheostomy are 2 respiratory therapies in widespread use that offer life-saving therapeutic options for care in and out of hospitals. Both types of respiratory technology require continued usage and thus are a source of constant pressure placing the patient at high risk for hospital-acquired pressure injuries (HAPI), especially when they are in an altered medical state of health. This article describes evidence-based practice changes aimed to decrease pressure injury related to these 2 devices.

All authors certify that they have no financial or commercial conflict of interest associated with the subject matter written about in this article. All authors also have no funding sources outside of their place of employment.

[a] Department of Nursing, Children's Hospital of Philadelphia, 3401 Civic Center Boulevard, Main 8S41, Philadelphia, PA 19104, USA; [b] Department of Nursing, Children's Hospital of Philadelphia, 3401 Civic Center Boulevard, Main A282, Philadelphia, PA 19104, USA; [c] Department of Nursing, Children's Hospital of Philadelphia, 3401 Civic Center Boulevard, Main 7 NE (PCU), Philadelphia, PA 19104, USA; [d] Department of Nursing, Children's Hospital of Philadelphia, 3401 Civic Center Boulevard, Main Hospital A282, Philadelphia, PA 19104, USA
* Corresponding author.
E-mail address: miske@email.chop.edu

Background

The National Pressure Ulcer Advisory Panel (NPUAP) defines a pressure injury as "localized damage to the skin and/or underlying soft tissue usually over a bony prominence or related to a medical or other device."[1] Pressure injuries, previously referred to as pressure ulcers, bed sores, and decubitus ulcers, are the result of pressure to tissue over time. The prevention of pressure injuries is important for many reasons. Pressure injuries can cause the following:

- Patient pain and discomfort
- Temporary or permanent disfigurement
- Potentially life-threatening infection
- Need for surgical debridement or reconstruction
- Increased length of stay (LOS)

In addition to the negative implications of pressure injury to the patient, there are negatives for the facility. There are increased costs to the hospital, including the rental of specialty beds, wound care supplies, nursing time, and increased LOS. Since October 2008, HAPI has been included in a list of hospital-acquired conditions not reimbursed by Medicare and Medicaid.[2] Many facilities participate in pressure injury surveillance and report to benchmarking agencies, such as National Database of Nursing Quality Indicators or Solutions for Patient Safety (SPS); comparing the rate to other facilities' rates serves as an external motivator for improvement. At the Children's Hospital of Philadelphia (CHOP), a 500-bed, tertiary-care, free-standing children's hospital and health network, stage 3, stage 4, and unstageable injuries are reported to SPS and are referred to as "reportable," differentiating them from partial-thickness injuries such as stage 1 and stage 2.

The terminology used to describe the extent of tissue damage from a pressure injury is standardized using the staging system from the NPUAP (**Table 1**).

One tends to think of occipital injury in smaller children and sacral injury in older children and adults when one thinks of pressure injury. However, one published study showed that 75% of HAPI were from devices, not from immobility. This same study demonstrated a baseline occurrence rate for tracheostomy-related pressure injuries of 8.1%.[3] In technology-dependent patients, the challenge to reduce pressure and time exposed to pressure is a barrier to pressure injury prevention given that some medical devices are life-sustaining and therefore must remain in place at all times.

Medical device–related pressure injury (MDRPI), including respiratory device–related HAPI, is staged using the NPUAP pressure injury staging system (see **Table 1**). Because the nose has very little depth of tissue between the surface of the skin and the underlying bone and cartilage, full-thickness pressure injuries can quickly advance to stage 4. Injuries that occur on mucus membranes such as the inside of the nares (from nasal prongs, nasal endotracheal tube, nasogastric tubes, and so forth) or at the tracheostomy stoma are identified as mucous membrane pressure injuries. The tissue layers of mucus membranes are different from skin; therefore, these are staged differently using the term mucosal injury. They are not considered as reportable injuries at this time.

The overall prevalence (number of patients with injuries divided by number of patients surveyed) of MDRPI has been reported to be 3.1% of patients; the injuries in this study were identified at 3 to 13 days from application of the medical device.[4] At the authors' institution, pressure injury surveillance includes periodic prevalence surveys and ongoing incidence density data collection (**Figs. 1** and **2**). It should be noted

| Table 1 |
| Pressure injury staging definitions |

Pressure Injury Staging Definitions	
Stage 1 pressure injury	Nonblanchable erythema of intact skin
Stage 2 pressure injury	Partial-thickness skin loss with exposed epidermis, may present as an intact or ruptured serum-filled blister
Stage 3 pressure injury	Full-thickness skin loss in which fat is visible in the ulcer. The depth of tissue damage varies by anatomical location. Fascia, muscle, tendon, ligament, cartilage, and/or bone are not exposed
Stage 4 pressure injury	Full-thickness skin and tissue loss with exposed or directly palpable fascia, muscle, tendon, ligament cartilage, or bone in the ulcer
Unstageable pressure injury	Obscured full-thickness skin and tissue loss in which the extent of the tissue damage within the ulcer cannot be confirmed because it is obscured by slough or eschar
Deep tissue pressure injury	Persistent nonblanchable deep red, maroon, or purple discoloration
Mucosal membrane pressure injury	Mucosal membrane pressure injury is found on mucous membranes with a history of a medical device in use at the location of the injury. Due to the anatomy of the tissue these injuries cannot be staged

From National Pressure Ulcer Advisory Panel (NPUAP) announces a change in terminology from pressure ulcer to pressure injury and updates the stages of pressure injury. Available at: www.npuap.org/national-pressure-ulcer-advisory-panel-npuap-announces-a-change-in-terminology-from-pressure-ulcer-to-pressure-injury-and-updates-the-stages-of-pressure-injury. Accessed May 30, 2016; with permission.

that a new method of collecting HAPI incidence was initiated in March 2015 with a subsequent increase in stage 1 and 2 HAPIs reported.

These data mirror what has been reported in the literature: 71% of HAPI at the authors' institution are MDRPI (**Fig. 3**). Further breakdown of the data demonstrates that respiratory devices such as NIPPV and tracheostomy are 2 major contributors to MDRPI at CHOP (**Fig. 4**). What follows is a discussion of those challenges and the authors' approach to improving practice.

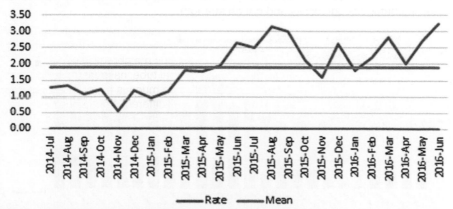

Fig. 1. HAPI incidence density per 1000 patient-days (all stages).

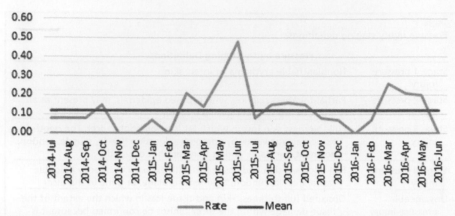

Fig. 2. HAPI incidence density per 1000 patient-days (stage 3, 4, and unstageable).

NONINVASIVE POSITIVE PRESSURE VENTILATION
History

Noninvasive ventilation became widespread between the 1930s and 1950s as a result of the polio epidemic.[5] At that time, patients with polio were placed into a cylinder enclosing their body below the neck. The cylinder used electrical power to create a negative pressure environment within the cylinder, in order to mimic the effort of the diaphragm, to promote air entry into the lungs. Expiration continued to be a passive process. In the 1980s, the technology changed to create a tabletop machine that would produce positive pressure airflow into the lungs of a patient via an interface that connected the patient to the machine tubing. It was not intended for 24 hour per /day use, but rather as a treatment for sleep apnea.[6]

Patients using NIPPV have conditions ranging from obstructive sleep apnea, neurologic impairment, control of breathing disorders, and chronic lung disease.[7] Like invasive ventilation (via endotracheal tube or tracheostomy tube), NIPPV can be used with patients of all ages and diagnoses except facial trauma or burns and offers advantages from a medical perspective. There is no surgery required to use NIPPV. The ventilator can be the same as one used for invasive ventilation, which is sensitive to the patient's respiratory demands and portable for use outside of a hospital environment. NIPPV preserves the body's ability to warm, filter, and humidify air as well as preserving natural cough ability and cough strength.

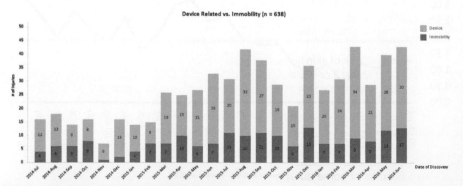

Fig. 3. Immobility versus device-related HAPI.

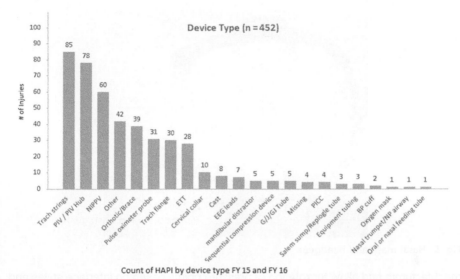

Count of HAPI by device type FY 15 and FY 16

Fig. 4. CHOP HAPI by device. BP, blood pressure; EEG, electroencephalogram; Trach, tracheotomy.

Use of this technology has grown exponentially in the past 20 years, and more indications for use ranging from neonatal intensive care unit (NICU) postextubation to pediatric intensive care unit avoiding intubation appear regularly.[8,9] The pulmonary medicine division at an east coast tertiary care children's hospital has experienced an increase in patients using NIPPV from 33% of their technology-dependent patients in 1999 to 59% in 2016. These numbers exclude patients followed by the Sleep Medicine program and are nearly evenly divided with 136 patients using continuous positive airway pressure and 148 using BiLevel positive airway pressure in 2016. When data were initially tracked for skin injury prevalence at this institution in 2010, it was discovered that NIPPV was the number one medical device causing skin injury.[10]

Skin Injury from Noninvasive Positive Pressure Ventilation

Because NIPPV requires constant pressure for up to 24 hours per day over areas with little to no subcutaneous fat, the risk for HAPI is high.[11–13] In some reports, NIPPV is responsible for a 10% to 20% incidence of HAPI.[9,14] The nasal bridge is an area with particular vulnerability to skin injury, and nasal injury can occur in up to 40% of infants using NIPPV.[12] The forehead, cheek, cartilage of ear, back of neck, and occiput are also impacted by the pressure points of the interface and headgear (**Fig. 5**), and different institutions have different areas of vulnerability in regard to skin injury from NIPPV.[15]

Because of the lack of skin layers, an area of nonblanchable redness (stage 1 injury) can progress to stage 3 or worse in a very short period of time (in the authors' institution, they have seen this occur in a 12-hour period). Because of the size of infant and pediatric patients, an area of skin injury affecting interface placement can have a high impact on ability to use this type of respiratory support because there may not be alternative interfaces available to relieve pressure from that area.

Interface Options

No single hospital or home durable medical equipment company is able to stock and dispense all available interfaces, but choices increase on a regular basis from

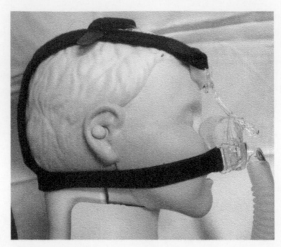

Fig. 5. Nasal mask and headgear.

manufacturers and allow for rotation of pressure points based on interface styles and patient preference. Internet sites offer more than 22 manufacturers of NIPPV interfaces and 100 styles, sizes, and colors of NIPPV interfaces, ranging from nasal prongs, to nasal mask, oral, full face mask, or a hybrid version that incorporates features from more than one interface type. The material used for these interfaces and their cushions can be silicone, gel, plastic, fabric, or foam. Interface material is not able to be customized; each manufacturer designs an interface with a set material. Patient preference and interface fit[16] determine "best" choices. There is lack of evidence in the literature regarding interface material known to produce more or less pressure injuries.

METHODS
Change Process: One Hospital's Evidence-Based Practice Journey to Implement Noninvasive Positive Pressure Ventilation–Related Hospital-Acquired Pressure Injuries Prevention

Periodic procedure review, in order to comply with various state and national regulatory agencies, is required. Depending on the patient population of a hospital, this can be a compendium of smaller unit-based groups or a multidisciplinary hospital-wide workgroup. However, each specialty area will have a vested interest in preserving unit-based culture. Use of an evidence-based practice (EBP) methodology to guide performance and provide methods of tests of change helps to minimize staff preference and provides objectivity.[17] Hospital value analysis teams also influence final determination of any changes in product selection. In today's health care economy, value analysis of products determines continued use and a true EBP approach dictates modifications based on this analysis.[18]

Two nurses from the inpatient pulmonary unit identified skin injury prevention as a goal for patients receiving NIPPV in 2008. The Certified Wound Ostomy Continence Nurse Practitioner (CWOC-NP) at the hospital convened a project team, due to nurses in the NICU simultaneously meeting to discuss skin injury prevention in neonates. The team was created in 2009 with interested members of the respiratory and nursing staff who cared for patients receiving NIPPV, the pulmonary clinical nurse specialist (CNS), CWOC-NP, and nurse researcher. In 2011, literature reviews and hospital benchmarking resulted in revisions to the hospital's nursing standard and procedure for NIPPV, in order to prevent HAPIs from this medical device.

Besides standardized assessments, a new silicone-based foam product was intro-duced to be placed under the NIPPV interface. Multiple thicknesses and types of the foam product were required to meet the needs of all patient types, from neonate to young adult. Mandatory training in the form of a written learning module and interac-tive simulation occurred, over a 5-month period, for all staff in the units who care for patients with NIPPV. The simulation was performed by 2 bedside caregivers with facil-itation by project team members to apply the concepts and new education from the revised nursing standard: correctly sizing an NIPPV interface, applying a foam dres-sing product between the interface and the skin, collaborating for skin assessment, and changing the interface based on assessment findings or identified time limits. Staff required coaching to correctly size the foam dressing, because the tendency was to cut it the same size as the interface. If it was not cut larger than the interface, the dressing relocated with any interface movement, increasing the chance of aspira-tion or airway occlusion under the interface. Customized templates were recommen-ded to be at each bedside for padding of all pressure points under the interface.

HOSPITAL-ACQUIRED PRESSURE INJURIES PREVENTION PRACTICE CHANGES FOR NONINVASIVE POSITIVE PRESSURE VENTILATION

The following practice changes occurred regarding standardized assessments and interface placement as a result of the EBP efforts. Anyone providing care for a patient using NIPPV needs to be aware of the areas of concern for HAPI and continually eval-uate the patient and the interface to prevent skin injury. Formal assessment includes removal of the interface with skin appraisal at all pressure points every 4 hours.[16,19] Assessments made at each appraisal include the following:

- Interface edges should not touch the epicanthal fold or upper lip
- Nasal mask material should not press against outer portion of nares
- Observe for conjunctival or nasal irritation
- Interface material should not be compressed
- Cheeks should not be visibly indented
- One to 2 fingers should fit under straps holding interface
- Nasal prongs should slide into nares, not push nostrils out
- Distal end of nose should not be flattened or pushed back toward face
- Interface should be centered on nose/face

Squires and Hyndman[19] published a literature review of injuries related to nasal continuous positive airway pressure for the extremely low-birth-weight infant. Their findings for prevention can apply to any form of NIPPV because the best intervention is prevention. All of these clinical guidelines were included in the revision to the nursing standard of care for patients using NIPPV:

- Use the smallest interface possible
- Use skin barrier for all patients
- Use 2 providers to apply interface unless patient is able to assist, so as to keep centered
- Affix tubing from machine to interface after interface and headgear are in place
- Tighten the headgear straps slowly, if needed, to minimize (not eliminate) leak
- Use a chin strap or pacifier to minimize leak from oral cavity
- Airflow from exhalation ports is to be expected—direct away from eyes

In an effort to have unit staff "own" the practice changes instituted, the CWOC-NP developed a program for each unit to identify a subgroup of nurses to receive additional education in skin injury prevention. These unit-based skin champions offer expertise at the front line: help colleagues troubleshoot skin-related concerns, confirm and stage suspected pressure injuries, perform monthly audits, participate in prevalence surveys and develop unit-based education to increase compliance with the standard of care, and decrease the incidence of skin injury from all causes.

OUTCOMES RELATED TO NONINVASIVE POSITIVE PRESSURE VENTILATION PRACTICE CHANGES

The Children's Hospital Association (CHA) has instituted standardized metrics for its member hospitals in order to improve performance.[15] Each year a target is set with initial reporting done quarterly; many institutions perform a monthly skin survey to analyze incidence. On the pulmonary inpatient unit of an east coast children's hospital, the Fiscal Year (FY) 2015 rate for NIPPV-related HAPI events was less than that of FY 2016; however, events of reportable harm did not occur in either year on this unit (**Table 2**). The increase in patient days and staff turnover impact the feasibility of sustained improvement, even in a unit that sees these patients on a routine basis. For that reason, there continues to be a unit-based focus on data collection and quality improvement related to NIPPV.

The intensive care areas of the same hospital compared with the pulmonary unit reported more HAPI events on the monthly skin injury surveys, as displayed in **Fig. 6**. As described by Peterson and colleagues,[15] patients with cardiac or respiratory instability are at higher risk for development of HAPIs based on the presence of immobility, poor perfusion, nutritional deficiency, or edema. The hospital as a whole experienced an increase in volume and acuity in FY 16, which may have contributed to the overall increase in HAPIs.

A children's hospital on the west coast created an interdisciplinary team to join the CHA collaborative and implement organizational changes.[15] Their initial efforts demonstrated an increase in injuries reported (3.3/1000 patient-days), consistent with increased awareness, followed by decreased HAPIs after 6 months (1.9/1000 patient-days). Occurrences again increased to 3/1000 patient-days 6 months later (2011). They redesigned their hospital-based team and, led by the CNS, accomplished a 67% reduction in reportable HAPIs (n = 3) in a 1-year period and a 60% reduction in reportable injuries during the 4-year interventional period.[15]

The results from these 2 institutions highlight the difficulty in sustaining improvement results in patients who require NIPPV. Similar challenges exist when considering tracheostomy- and tracheostomy securement device-related HAPIs.

Table 2
Pulmonary unit noninvasive positive pressure ventilation hospital-acquired pressure injury incidence

Pulmonary Unit NIPPV HAPI Incidence	FY 15	FY 16
No. of NIPPV patients	456	573
NIPPV days	2789	3423
Incidence rate (per 1000 NIPPV patient-days)	1.79	2.04
Total patient-days	7735	8115
Incidence rate (per 1000 patient-days)	0.64	0.86

Data from Children's Hospital of Philadelphia, Philadelphia. July 1, 2014 to June 30, 2016.

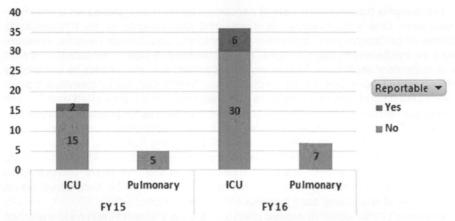

Fig. 6. Count of NIPPV-related HAPIs. ICU, intensive care unit.

TRACHEOSTOMY
History

Incidence of pediatric tracheostomy has increased over the last few decades, with about 4900 pediatric tracheostomies performed in the United States every year.[20] Fifty years ago, pediatric tracheostomy was mostly considered an emergency procedure to address airway obstruction from acute infections such as croup, epiglottitis, and diphtheria.[21,22] These children required short-term ventilation while the infectious process resolved and were generally decannulated after surviving the acute episode.[20] Common indications for today's pediatric tracheostomies have shifted dramatically. Medical advances have resulted in increased survival of premature neonates and those with complex cardiopulmonary disease, who may require long-term mechanical ventilation.[21] Tracheostomy is now performed more frequently in infants, especially premature infants, and children with chronic conditions.[21,23] The most common primary indication for tracheostomy is cardiopulmonary disease, which accounted for just 13% of tracheostomies in 1984 and now accounts for almost 40%.[22] Other common indications include neurologic impairment, airway obstruction, craniofacial abnormalities, and traumatic injury.[22]

Not only are there nearly 5000 new tracheostomies performed each year in the United States, but hospitalizations of children with pre-existing tracheostomies are also substantial in number. Using the Healthcare Cost and Utilization Project Kids' Inpatient Database, Zhu and colleagues[23] identified 21,541 hospitalizations of children with pre-existing tracheostomies in 2009. Complexity of this patient population was illustrated in this review, with children on average having 5 chronic conditions.[23]

Literature Review

Skin injury from tracheostomies and tracheostomy securement devices

The NPUAP has defined Best Practices for Prevention of Medical Device-Related Pressure Ulcers in Pediatric Populations.[24] These Best Practices include inspecting the skin in contact with the device at least daily; being aware of edema under devices and potential for skin breakdown; and cushioning and protecting the skin with dressings in high-risk areas. The NPUAP recommends that staff be educated on correct use of devices and prevention of skin breakdown. The literature also promotes that patients and their families be taught to identify tracheostomy-related skin breakdown.[3,25,26]

The complex tracheostomy patient population poses many challenges during hospitalization. One such challenge is maintaining skin integrity at the tracheostomy stoma, at peristomal skin, and under tracheostomy securement devices. Pressure from the tracheostomy tube, flanges, and securement devices; moisture from sweat and respiratory secretions; friction and shear forces; and the inability to completely offload pressure or rotate the device place the patient at high risk for developing pressure ulcers. In addition, many patients with tracheostomies have limited mobility and neurologic responsiveness, which further increase their risk for pressure injury development.[3] The literature has placed little emphasis on tracheostomy-related skin complications. When these complications are addressed, the focus has been on stomal complications mostly in the immediate postoperative period.[27–30] Although patients are at high risk for wound-healing complications in the immediate postoperative period, the risk for development of a pressure injury should be considered on an ongoing basis and during each subsequent hospitalization.

Incidence of tracheostomy-related pressure ulcers is unclear in the literature and has been reported between 0% and 39%, with a higher incidence noted in the infant population.[29,31] One challenge in determining accurate incidence is the inconsistent application of the NPUAP staging system to tracheostomy-related injuries, with several studies not using the staging system to classify these wounds.[27,29,31] In addition, there may be a general underrepresentation of tracheostomy-related pressure ulcers being reported. One study attempted to look at historical data to determine effectiveness of a new intervention, but found that although 10 patients (38.5%) who underwent tracheostomy during the 10-month study period had a postoperative tracheostomy-related wound, a total of 5 such injuries were captured in medical records in the 5 years before the start of the study.[28] They attributed this to incomplete documentation and lack of appreciation for prevalence and significance of these wounds.[28]

Lack of Consensus in the Literature

Tracheostomy tube type

Some studies have found that the type of tracheostomy tube used impacts the incidence of tracheostomy-related pressure injuries at the stoma. Boesch and colleagues[3] noted less injury with tracheostomy tubes with a flexible extension separating the flanges from the 15-mm adapter, and flanges at a 30% angle to conform to the neck contours of an infant or young child. Jaryszak and colleagues[29] noted that use of a tracheostomy tube with a flexible extension was more predictive of wound development than use of other tubes.

Neck protectants

There is no consensus for type of dressing to be used at the stoma or under tracheostomy securement devices. Although gauze is the most commonly used barrier between the tracheostomy flange or ties and the patient's skin, various studies have looked at using different dressings to prevent pressure injuries. These dressings include solid pectin-based barriers, and plain or silver-impregnated silicone dressings.[3,27,30] One article recommends different types of stomal dressings depending on the amount of secretions, presence of skin breakdown, or presence of infection.[25] These dressings included gauze, polyurethane foam, hydrocolloid, silicone foam, carboxymethylcellulose impregnated with ionic silver, and nylon impregnated with silver.[25]

Tracheostomy Securement Device Tightness and Change Frequency

Recommendations for appropriate tracheostomy securement device tightness and frequency of change are often vague. Recommendations range from "only 1 finger fitting between the tie and the neck,"[25] to "only 1 loose or 2 snug finger-widths,"[32] to "ties should be tighter (in children) allowing only 1 finger, but remains comfortable."[33] Recommendations for frequency of tracheostomy securement device changes are that they should be replaced as needed according to facility-specific policy.[25]

METHODS
Change Process: One Hospital's Evidence-Based Practice Journey to Implement Tracheostomy-Related Hospital-Acquired Pressure Injuries Prevention

Description of population
The Progressive Care Unit (PCU) is a 24-bed inpatient tracheostomy/ventilator unit within a large pediatric hospital and serves as a bridge between intensive care and home or long-term care. Tracheostomy-related injuries account for most HAPI that occur in the PCU. These injuries are seen in 3 distinct areas: lateral and posterior neck from tracheostomy securement devices; anterior neck from tracheostomy flanges; and at the stoma or peristomal skin due to tension from the tracheostomy tube and ventilator tubing. Of these causes, injuries related to tracheostomy securement devices are the most common. In FY 2015, the PCU had a total of 35 pressure injuries, about half of which were caused by tracheostomy securement devices (n = 17). A multipronged improvement approach has resulted in some success in decreasing the incidence of tracheostomy securement device-related HAPIs in the PCU. This approach included staff education and engagement; recruitment and training of Skin Champions; patient/family education; skin rounds; and clinical practice changes.

Staff Education and Engagement
Staff engagement has been essential in implementing improvement efforts and clinical practice changes. Education has been disseminated to staff using various modalities including an online learning module, lectures, inclusion of pressure injury prevention in the unit orientation checklist, article reviews, and discussions at staff meetings.

To address staff turnover and ensure that new nursing staff receives education on pressure injury prevention and treatment, all new nurse hires in the PCU receive a lecture on respiratory device–related pressure injuries, presented by the unit-based CNS. This lecture reviews unit data, basics on staging, preventative measures, and treatment options. The acronym "PREVENTT" is used to highlight preventative measures specifically related to tracheostomy flanges and securement devices (**Fig. 7**). In addition to this lecture, pressure injury prevention has been added to the unit's orientation checklist to ensure that preceptors review available resources and unit best practices with all new hires.

Ensuring that staff is aware of pressure injury incidence and trends on the unit has also been important. Staff awareness has been accomplished with visual displays on the unit, inclusion of data in the unit newsletter, and presentation of data at unit-based Shared Governance meetings.

In addition to ensuring that all nursing staff receives basic education on the prevention, identification, and treatment of pressure injuries, there is a smaller group of nurses that have received additional training in skin-related issues, with a heavy emphasis on pressure injury prevention. These Skin Champions have been essential in unit-based improvement efforts. Skin Champions offer expertise at the front line to help colleagues troubleshoot skin-related concerns and confirm and stage suspected pressure injuries. In addition, Skin Champions perform monthly audits, participate in monthly prevalence surveys, and create and disseminate education to staff.

PREVENTT

Tracheostomy-related Pressure Injuries

Partner with caregivers

- On admission, ask if patient has a history of skin injury under trach device or trach ties
- Explain risk of skin injury and encourage caregivers to report any redness or breakdown
- Explain that plan of care may need to be different while patient is in the hospital

Reduce friction with neck protectant

- No-sting barrier film under ties for all patients ($\geq$1 mo) without breakdown or erythema
- Mepilex lite under ties for blanchable erythema
- Mepilex under ties for pressure injuries (blanchable erythema, blister, open area, DTI)
- Dressing under ties should be visible 1–2 cm above and below the ties
- Stoma dressing should be large enough to protect stoma *and* skin under flanges

Eliminate moisture

- Check often! Moisture can result from sweat, secretions, baths, emesis, feeding
- Change wet ties and dressings as soon as possible
- For excessive moisture or ties requiring multiple changes: contact ENT and Wound Care to explore other dressing options, and discuss options to decrease secretions with front line ordering provider

Visualize skin under ties on admission & every 12h

- On admission, identify any pre-existing skin injury and document on initial EPIC assessment
- Notify front line ordering provider of any injuries present on admission
- Assess neck under ties/flanges once per shift (every 12 h)

EPIC Documentation

- String skin alteration check, neck protectant on Respiratory flowsheet
- Any abnormalities in neck assessment noted in Minor Skin Alterations (Trach Skin Alteration)
- If a pressure injury is present, add Pressure Ulcer LDA

Non-blanchable erythema is a Stage 1 pressure injury

- Document as a pressure injury (add Pressure Ulcer in LDAs)
- Use Mepilex lite to protect from additional friction and moisture

Ties loose enough to slip one finger comfortably between ties and neck

- Some patients may require looser application
- Balance between too tight that causes breakdown and too loose that increases decannulation risk

Treatment

- Every pressure injury needs a formal treatment plan to prevent progression and promote healing
- Collaborate with CNS, Skin Champ, or WOCN to establish treatment plan

Fig. 7. PREVENTT acronym.

Nursing and Medical Leadership Engagement

The unit-based CNS and Quality and Patient Safety Coordinator have led the PCU's pressure injury prevention improvement work, with support from the unit's Nursing and Respiratory Leadership teams and the hospital's Wound Care program. This partnership has been ideal, as the CNS lends clinical expertise and the Quality and Patient Safety Coordinator helps coordinate rapid improvement cycles and aids in analysis of data. A workgroup dedicated to reducing tracheostomy-related pressure injuries now offers additional support for the implementation of quality improvement projects and practice changes and includes the unit's Respiratory Clinical Specialist, Respiratory Quality and Patient Safety Coordinator, and an enterprise Improvement Advisor. Current pressure injuries and plans for treatment are discussed during morning rounds with the multidisciplinary team. HAPIs are a standing topic at monthly Nursing Leadership meetings, and injuries are also presented on a quarterly basis to attendings, fellows, and nurse practitioners.

Patient and Family Education

In the PCU, a need was identified to increase family involvement in both the prevention and the identification of pressure injuries. Many PCU patients' families are intimately involved in the care of their children and may identify early subtle changes in their children's skin that may precipitate a pressure injury. The hospital's Pressure Ulcer Prevention patient/family education sheet is reviewed with families and used to educate them about risks, preventative measures, and treatment options. In addition, posters are displayed at each bedside, which includes pictures of the various devices that can cause pressure injuries and ways families can partner with the health care team to prevent device-related pressure injuries.

Skin Rounds

The unit-based CNS and the nurse or nurse practitioner from the Wound Care program conduct weekly rounds on the unit. Skin Rounds are an opportunity to address current skin issues, provide just-in-time education to nursing staff, and implement injury prevention strategies for at-risk patients. Recommendations are made and, in collaboration with the medical team, treatment interventions are ordered when needed.

HOSPITAL-ACQUIRED PRESSURE INJURIES PREVENTION PRACTICE CHANGES FOR TRACHEOSTOMY

Skin Assessment Under Tracheostomy Securement Devices

A thorough assessment of skin around the tracheostomy tube and under securement devices is important so early changes in skin integrity can be detected and addressed before progression to a pressure injury occurs. The hospital's Nursing Standard already stated that skin under securement devices should be assessed, but did not specify frequency of assessments or how to perform a thorough assessment. Without specific guidance, staff often assessed skin under the securement device by moving the securement device slightly in an attempt to visualize the skin underneath. Few injuries were identified using this method, with most injuries identified on days when the securement devices were due to be changed—a time when ties were unfastened and a thorough assessment was performed. A quality-improvement project was initiated in the PCU to trial shiftly assessment of the neck skin and folds with complete unfastening of securement devices. This practice allowed a thorough assessment of the neck and temporary off-loading of the constant pressure from the devices.

Neck Protectant Under Tracheostomy Securement Devices

The PCU has implemented a standardization of practice to ensure that all patients receive a protective barrier between their neck and the tracheostomy securement device. Film-forming barriers help protect skin from moisture and friction.[34] As a preventative practice, a film-forming barrier is applied to patients' necks that show no signs of skin breakdown. If blanchable erythema is noted under securement devices, use of a thin silicone foam dressing to provide cushioning and protection from friction is considered. If a pressure injury is noted, care is escalated to a thicker silicone foam dressing to provide additional cushioning; a silver-impregnated foam dressing may be considered for its antimicrobial properties. It is important to note that all dressings should be changed when wet or soiled, because moisture against the skin can further compromise skin integrity and contribute to the development of a pressure injury or impact the healing process of an existing injury.

Securement Device Tightness

The hospital implemented securement device tightness checks, completed by respiratory therapists every 4 hours. This addition was made to address concerns that factors such as fluid shifts could influence the tightness of securement devices throughout the day. The authors' hospital uses language similar to that in the literature, recommending that the clinician checking tightness be able to fit one finger securely under the securement device.

Securement Device Change Frequency

The hospital's Nursing Standard currently states that securement devices should be changed 3 times per week and more frequently if the securement devices become wet or soiled. After benchmarking with several other institutions, the PCU trialed daily securement device changes. As with the shiftly neck skin assessments, this offered an opportunity for temporary off-loading of the pressure produced by the securement device and allowed nurses and respiratory therapists to complete a thorough assessment of the neck skin and folds. In addition, providing a new securement device daily helps address moisture management concerns for diaphoretic patients or those with copious secretions.

OUTCOMES RELATED TO TRACHEOSTOMY PRACTICE CHANGES

Standardizing the frequency of neck assessments under tracheostomy securement devices and the method for performing these assessments has shown promising improvement in the incidence of securement device-related pressure injuries. Tracheostomy securement device-related pressure injuries in the PCU decreased after the implementation of shiftly neck assessments, with the 4 months following the practice change being injury free (**Fig. 8**). The improvement was not sustained, however, and incidence began to increase again over time. Moreover, when the practice was applied hospital-wide, the results were not replicated and incidence of tracheostomy securement device-related pressure injuries increased.

Implementation of daily securement device changes also demonstrated promising results in reducing pressure injuries (**Fig. 9**). The authors continue to monitor incidence and rate to determine if the improvement will be sustained.

DISCUSSION

Hospital staff has a direct impact on the prevention of HAPI related to respiratory support technology. As they initiate the respiratory support therapy and prepare caregivers for home, they need to be aware of measures that influence the success of the therapy, in terms of effectiveness and compliance, as well as skin preservation.[11,17] Ultimately, staff and caregiver vigilance is essential to prevent HAPI in patients who require respiratory support devices.

None of the interventions at the authors' institution have proven to be a "magic bullet" for the prevention of HAPIs related to NIPPV or tracheostomy and tracheostomy securement device–related pressure ulcers; patients continue to be harmed each

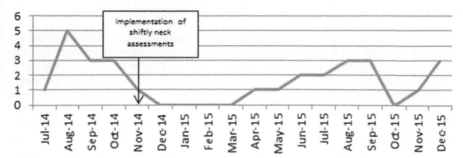

Fig. 8. Tracheostomy securement device-related HAPI in the PCU.

month. It is possible that increased awareness among staff hospital-wide may have led to increased reporting. Additional quality improvement efforts and subsequent practice changes continue to address these issues. In addition, the tracheostomy decannulation rates are continually and carefully monitored to ensure that the HAPI prevention practice changes are not associated with an increase in potentially life-threatening dislodgements.

Some patients seem to be more susceptible to injury, as several "repeat offenders" have been identified who continue to develop injuries despite improvement efforts. Bedside reviews have been conducted to try to identify trends that may indicate that a patient is at higher risk of developing an injury, without reliable results. An NPUAP best practice in the prevention of device-related pressure ulcers is to avoid placement of the device over sites of prior existing pressure injuries.[24] Avoidance of sites of prior pressure injuries is not possible when dealing with tracheostomy and securement device-related pressure ulcers, as these patients require these devices 24 hours per day and there is no opportunity for rotating to a different device. Likewise, rotation of interface may not be possible for some patients who require NIPPV, and intubation may need to be an alternative. More research is needed to help identify preventative measures for these challenging patient populations.

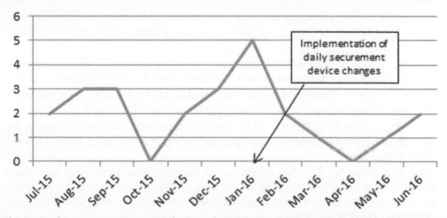

Fig. 9. Tracheostomy securement device-related pressure injuries in the PCU. Note: Some patients did not receive daily securement device changes during the trial period due to patient-specific factors. Patients who developed a pressure injury but were not receiving daily securement device changes were not included in this chart.

SUMMARY

Safe delivery of therapeutic respiratory support requires all staff involved to understand the necessity of the respiratory therapy, comprehend the mechanism of pressure injury development, and recognize the ability they have to prevent skin injury. In an effort to deliver evidenced-based care, on-going research is needed to identify best practices, implement them, and sustain their use. In order to implement changes on a hospital-wide level, staff education is necessary to increase staff awareness, competence, and knowledge. Sustainability requires constant vigilance in the form of regular and timely assessments, unit-based rounding, and consistent quality improvement efforts along with transparency of compliance with hospital standards and procedures to prevent HAPI's.

REFERENCES

1. National Pressure Ulcer Advisory Panel (NPUAP) announces a change in terminology from pressure ulcer to pressure injury and updates the stages of pressure injury. Available at: www.npuap.org/national-pressure-ulcer-advisory-panel-npuap-announces-a-change-in-terminology-from-pressure-ulcer-to-pressure-injury-and-updates-the-stages-of-pressure-injury. Accessed May 30, 2016.
2. Centers for Medicare & Medicaid Services Hospital Acquired Conditions. Available at: https://www.cms.gov/Medicare/Medicare-Fee-for-Service-Payment/HospitalAcqCond/index.html?redirect=/hospitalacqcond/06_hospital-acquired_conditions.asp. Accessed July 22, 2016.
3. Boesch R, Myers C, Dressman K, et al. Prevention of tracheostomy-related pressure ulcers in children. Pediatrics 2012;129(3):e792–7.
4. Coyer F, Stotts N, Blackman V. A prospective window into medical device-related pressure ulcers in intensive care. Int Wound J 2014;11(6):656–64. Available at: MEDLINE with Full Text, Ipswich, MA. Accessed June 30, 2016.
5. Meduri GU, Hill N. Noninvasive positive pressure ventilation in patients with acute respiratory failure. Clin Chest Med 1996;17:513–53.
6. Mehta S, Hill NS. Noninvasive ventilation. Am J Respir Crit Care Med 2001;163(2): 540–77.
7. Fauroux B, Boffa C, Desguerre I, et al. Long-term noninvasive mechanical ventilation for children at home: a national survey. Pediatr Pulmonol 2003;35(2): 119–25.
8. Joshi G, Tobias JD. A five-year experience with the use of BiPAP in a pediatric intensive care unit population. J Intensive Care Med 2007;22(1):38–43.
9. Cavari Y, Sofer S, Rozovski U, et al. Non invasive positive pressure ventilation in infants with respiratory failure. Pediatr Pulmonol 2012;47:1019–25.
10. Miske LJ, Hickey EM, Stellar J, et al. Hospital acquired skin injury related to the use of noninvasive positive pressure ventilation. Chest 2012;142(4_Meeting Abstracts):772A.
11. Yong SC, Chen SJ, Boo NY. Incidence of nasal trauma associated with nasal prong versus nasal mask during continuous positive airway pressure treatment in very low birthweight infants: a randomised control study. Arch Dis Child Fetal Neonatal Ed 2005;90:F480–3.
12. Buettker V, Hug MI, Baenziger O, et al. Advantages and disadvantages of different nasal CPAP systems in newborns. Intensive Care Med 2004;30(5): 926–30.

13. Robertson NJ, McCarthy LS, Hamilton PA, et al. Nasal deformities resulting from flow driver continuous positive airway pressure. Arch Dis Child Fetal Neonatal Ed 1996;75:F209–12.

14. Hill NS. Problems, remedies and strategies to optimize the success of noninvasive ventilation. In: Hill NS, editor. Noninvasive positive pressure ventilation: principles and applications. Armonk (NY): Futura Publishing Co, Inc; 2001. p. 169–85.

15. Peterson J, Adlard K, Walti BI, et al. Clinical nurse specialist collaboration to recognize, prevent and treat pediatric pressure ulcers. Clin Nurse Spec 2015; 29(5):276–82.

16. Teague GW, Lang DM. Application of NPPV in children. In: Hill NS, editor. Noninvasive positive pressure ventilation: principles and applications. Armonk (NY): Futura Publishing Co, Inc; 2001. p. 169–85.

17. Carter T. The application of the methods of evidence-based practice to occupational health. Occup Med 2000;50(4):231–6.

18. Gold MR, Siegel JE, Russell LB, et al, editors. Cost-effectiveness in health and medicine. Oxford (NY): Oxford University Press; 1996.

19. Squires A, Hyndman M. Prevention of nasal injuries secondary to NCPAP application in the ELBW infant. Neonatal Netw 2009;28(1):13–27.

20. Lewis CW, Carron JD, Perkins JA, et al. Tracheostomy in pediatric patients. Arch Otolaryngol Head Neck Surg 2003;129:523–9.

21. Funamura JL, Durbin-Johnson B, Tollefson TT, et al. Pediatric tracheostomy: indications and decannulation outcomes. Laryngoscope 2014;124:1952–8.

22. Gergin O, Adil EA, Kawai K, et al. Indications of pediatric tracheostomy over the last 30 years: has anything changed? Int J Pediatr Otorhinolaryngol 2016;87: 144–7.

23. Zhu H, Das P, Roberson DW, et al. Hospitalizations in children with preexisting tracheostomy: a national perspective. Laryngoscope 2015;125:462–8.

24. Best practices for prevention of medical device-related pressure ulcers in pediatric populations. National Pressure Ulcer Advisory Panel Web Site. 2013. Available at: http://www.npuap.org/wp-content/uploads/2013/04/BestPractices-Pediatric1.pdf. Accessed July 28, 2016.

25. Morris LL, Whitmer A, McIntosh E. Tracheostomy care and complications in the intensive care unit. Crit Care Nurse 2013;33(5):18–30.

26. Mitchell RB, Hussey HM, Setzen G, et al. Clinical consensus statement: tracheostomy care. Otolaryng Head Neck 2013;148(1):6–20.

27. Chuang W, Huang W, Chen M, et al. Gauze versus solid skin barrier for tracheostomy care: a crossover randomized clinical trial. J Wound Ostomy Cont 2013; 40(6):573–9.

28. Hartzell LD, Havens TN, Odom BH, et al. Enhanced tracheostomy wound healing using maltodextrin and sliver alginate compounds in pediatrics: a pilot study. Respir Care 2014;59(12):1857–62.

29. Jaryszak EM, Shah RK, Amling J, et al. Pediatric tracheostomy wound complications. Arch Otolaryngol 2011;137(4):363–6.

30. Kuo CY, Wootten CT, Tylor DA, et al. Prevention of pressure ulcers after pediatric tracheostomy using Mepilex Ag dressing. Laryngoscope 2013;123:3201–5.

31. Kremer B, Botos-Kremer AI, Eckel HE, et al. Indications, complications, and surgical techniques for pediatric tracheostomies—an update. J Pediatr Surg 2002; 37(11):1556–62.

32. Perry AG, Potter PA. Airway management: performing tracheostomy care. In: Epstein SR, editor. Clinical nursing skills and techniques. 6th edition. Philadelphia: Elsevier Mosby; 2006. p. 841–8.
33. Campisi P, Forte V. Pediatric tracheostomy. Semin Pediatr Surg 2016;25:191–5.
34. Lutz JB. Performance assessment of film forming barriers (skin sealants). St Paul (MN): 3M Health Care; 2002. Available at: http://multimedia.3m.com/mws/media/172627O/performance-assessment-of-film-forming-barriers.pdf.

Effective Management of Pain and Anxiety for the Pediatric Patient in the Emergency Department

Virginia B. Young, MSN, RN, PCNS-BC

KEYWORDS

- Pain • Anxiety • Pharmacologic • Nonpharmacologic • Emergency department (ED)
- Management • Pediatric

KEY POINTS

- There is suboptimal management of pain for children in the emergency department, although it has improved owing to research and increased knowledge of pediatric pain management.
- Barriers to adequate pain management have been identified in the literature.
- Assessment and reassessment of children's pain should occur using a validated tool that is appropriate for their age and cognitive level.
- Effective management of acute pain and anxiety in children should involve an approach that uses pharmacologic and nonpharmacologic interventions.
- The use of analgesics does not mask or delay diagnosis for the pediatric patient in the emergency department.

INTRODUCTION

Children present to the emergency department (ED) for a variety of painful conditions ranging from mild otitis to multisystem trauma. Oligoanalgesia or the inadequate treatment of pain[1] is common in the ED, and this can be particularly true for children.[2–4] Encouragingly, the trends for pain management in the ED are beginning to improve, largely owing to medical research, which has enhanced knowledge, and the dispelling of myths related to the pain experience in infants and children.[5,6] However, there remain barriers and gaps in the adequate management of pain for children in the ED.

Pain comes from the Latin word *poena* meaning penalty, retribution, or punishment and was once thought to be caused by evil humors or demons, or as a punishment from God.[7] Ancient methods of pain relief included measures such as religious

No disclosures.
Emergency Services, Children's Health, 1935 Medical District Drive, Dallas, TX 75235, USA
E-mail address: Ginger.young@childrens.com

Crit Care Nurs Clin N Am 29 (2017) 205–216
http://dx.doi.org/10.1016/j.cnc.2017.01.007
0899-5885/17/© 2017 Elsevier Inc. All rights reserved.

offerings, chanting as a diversion, the use of gongs or other noise making devices to frighten demons, electric eels laid on wounds, trepanning, and sucking out the pain with pipes.[7,8] Currently, a standard definition of pain is an unpleasant sensory sensation associated with actual or potential tissue damage.[9,10] Another well-accepted definition by McCaffery[11] is that "pain is whatever the experiencing person says it is, existing whenever the experiencing person says it does." In a joint statement, the American Academy of Pediatrics and the American Pain Society state that "pain is an inherently objective experience and should be assessed and treated as such."[12]

ETHICAL AND MORAL OBLIGATIONS FOR PAIN MANAGEMENT

Health care professionals (HCP) are obliged through ethical principles to provide pain relief and comfort to patients. In their ethics charter, the American Academy of Pain Medicine declares that physicians have an "ethical imperative" to provide relief from pain.[13] The International Association for the Study of Pain released a statement in the Declaration of Montreal declaring access to pain management as a basic human right, and that "withholding of pain treatment is profoundly wrong and leads to unnecessary suffering."[14] In a joint statement the American College of Emergency Physicians, the Emergency Nurses Association, the American Pain Society and the American Society of Pain Management Nursing state that "management of pain is an essential nursing and physician responsibility."[15]

BARRIERS TO ADEQUATE PAIN MANAGEMENT

Pain is a key reason why children present to the ED, and diagnostic testing and procedures may cause additional pain. Managing pain can be a challenge for even the most dedicated HCP. Studies have shown that children are a particularly vulnerable population when it comes to pain management, and are less likely to have their pain treated appropriately than adults.[12,16–18]

Emergency medicine providers commonly focus on the diagnosis or cause of the pain and may ignore the treatment of the pain itself.[3,19] Effective treatment of pediatric pain can be challenging and multiple studies have found there are disparities, and suboptimal management of pain for children in the ED.[16,20–22] Reports in the medical literature have identified barriers that often prevent adequate management of pain in children. Common barriers to effective pain management may be found in **Box 1**.

ASSESSMENT OF PAIN

Experts agree that the assessment and treatment of pain should occur rapidly. Studies have concluded that the immediate assessment, treatment, and attention to the patient's report of pain, or lack of improvement after an analgesic or intervention, are essential for successful pain management.[11,12,18] Because the ED is often the first encounter for children with painful illness or injuries, it is vital that pain be assessed and documented appropriately. In a study by Drendel and colleagues[16] that included more than 24,000 visits by children to EDs, it was found that only 44.5% of pediatric visits had documented pain scores. Visits categorized as a painful diagnosis had fewer than 60% of patients with pain scores documented (excluding pelvic pain), and for injuries known to be painful such as burns or orthopedic injuries the rate was about 50%.[16] Another study conducted in Illinois found that only 59% of children seen in EDs had a pain assessment documented.[24,25]

Children's pain is often underestimated because of a lack of appropriate assessment or belief that children cannot describe their pain.[7,26–28] The ability to indicate

---

Box 1
Common barriers to effective pain management

- Child's lack of understanding/cooperation and fear related to procedures
- Belief that children cannot adequately identify or describe their pain
- Lack of or inappropriate assessment or reassessment for pain
- The myth that children or infants do not feel pain or suffer less than adults
- Health care provider's fear of masking diagnosis with analgesics
- Fears of adverse effects from analgesics
- Belief that it will take too much time
- Health care provider's individual beliefs or values related to pain
- Lack of knowledge or application of treatment for pediatric pain
- Lack of resources to address pain in children

Data from Refs.[2,12,20,23]

---

the presence of pain has been found to be present as early as age 18 months.[12,29] Children as young as 18 months to 2 years begin to have words for pain and by the age of 3 some children can quantify their pain.[12,29]

Effective pain management begins with the ability to assess pain using an appropriate and validated tool. Several methods can be used to assess pain in children (**Table 1**). Self-report is considered the most reliable, but only if the child has the cognitive ability and the capacity for appropriate communication needed to describe or quantify their pain.[19,36] Substitution of a behavioral observation pain scale along with physiologic measurements is necessary for children and infants unable to report their own pain.[29,37]

Many validated self-report pain tools for children are available (see **Table 1**). Studies have shown that children can use self-report tools as early as ages 3 to 5, although children of that age may have difficulty knowing the difference between the experience of pain, and other distressing symptoms such as anxiety or nausea.[5] Most children greater than 8 years who are at a normal developmental level are able to use a self-report tool.[5]

Infants and children express pain through observable behaviors. Activities that can identify pain in infants and children are facial expressions, motor movement, and crying or verbalization.[29,37,38] Other behaviors that may indicate pain are body posture, change in muscle tone, and response to the environment.[6,37] Infants often express pain through harsh cries, and facial expressions such as lowered eyebrows that form a vertical furrow, bulge between brows with tightly closed eyes, and open mouth in a square shape.[6,37,38]

Behavioral observation tools are available for infants and young children and for those developmentally or cognitively unable to verbally report their pain, or are sedated (see **Table 1**).[29] In neonates and young infants, physiologic changes may also be noted with changes in vital signs such as heart rate, oxygen saturation, and palmar sweating.[38,39] Many premature infants cannot mount a response to pain and may be very still and passive.[38]

Pasero and McCaffery[37] developed a Hierarchy of Pain Assessment Techniques that may be used as a guide for assessments of patients, including infants and children, who are not able to verbalize their pain needs. The hierarchy begins with

Table 1
Pediatric pain assessment scales[a,b]

Behavioral Scales

Preterm to full term infants	Neonatal Infant Pain Scale (NIPS)	Evaluates 6 behaviors: facial expression breathing pattern, arm cry movement, leg movement, and state of arousal with a total score possible of 7, cry
Preterm to full-term infants	Premature Infant Pain Profile (PIPP)	Evaluates 7 indicators of pain, each on a 4-point scale: behavioral state, facial expression and physiologic changes heart rate, and oxygenation
0 mo to 7 y	Faces Legs Activity Cry Consolability (FLACC)	Evaluates 5 behaviors: facial expression, leg movement, activity, cry and consolability with a score ranging from 0–10

Self-report scales

Children ages 3–6 y	Pieces of Hurt (Poker Chip Tool)	Uses 4 poker chips that represent the amount of pain. Children use the quantity of chips to indicate how much they hurt
Children ages 4–17 y	FACES Pain Scale revised	Six faces each representing an increasing degree of pain from left to right. Scored 0, 2, 4, 6, 8, 10.
Children age 5 and older	Color Analog Scale	Wedge-shaped color gradate figure with a numbered scale on the other with a moveable slider.
Children ages 3–12 y	Oucher Scale	Two scales: a 0–100 numerical scale (if they can count to 100 by 1 or 10) for older children and 6 picture photographic scale for younger children

[a] This is not a comprehensive list of pediatric pain scales.
[b] These scales measure acute pain, which is a more common presentation for children in the emergency department.
Data from Refs.[30–35]

self-report, which is the preferred method of assessment. For the patient with limited verbal or cognitive abilities, this report may be a simple yes or no, or other physical cues may be used such as eye blinking or hand movement. Strategies in the hierarchy to aid pain assessments are as follows in preferred order: search for potential causes of pain, observe patient behaviors, use of behavioral pain tools, proxy reporting of pain, and analgesic trial.[37]

Search for Potential Causes of Pain

Identify any conditions or procedures that are likely to cause pain and treat accordingly.

Observe Patient Behaviors

Children exhibit specific behaviors in response to pain, including facial expressions, body or motor movement, crying or verbalization, body posture, and their response to the environment. Infants and children with chronic pain may not respond in the same manner because they may save energy by limiting their activity, withdrawing, and sleeping.

Use of Behavioral Pain Tools

There is no one tool that will meet the needs of all children. A tool should be chosen that has been validated for the specific age or needs of the child.

Proxy Reporting of Pain

Caregivers usually know their child's typical response to pain and can partner with the HCP in identifying behaviors that may supplement the pain assessment.

Analgesic Trial

If pain is suspected and the patient does not respond to their normal comfort measures an analgesic trial should be initiated using a nonopioid or low-dose opioid.[37] Whatever method of pain assessment is chosen, each emergency services area should have age-specific and cognitively appropriate tools available for the adequate assessment of pain in children. After treatment, reassessment should occur regularly to ensure adequate pain relief.[12] Remember, if it is painful for an adult it is painful for a child.

MANAGEMENT OF PAIN

In the ED, children may experience pain for a variety of reasons. Pain can be caused by acute illness or injury, trauma, recent surgery, or from medical procedures.[2–4] Some children also present with chronic pain. Studies have found that exposure to pain without adequate relief can have long-term consequences.[39,40] If pain is not addressed, it can cause fear and anxiety, and increase the child's perception of the severity of the pain they are experiencing.[40] Studies that include neonates and infants have found that untreated pain may cause permanent central nervous system changes and increased hypersensitivity to pain.[6,39,41] Near 6 months of age, some infants show signs that they have memory of painful procedures and children as young as 3 years have been found to have a recall of painful events.[41] This memory recall may be distorted negatively if the child was distressed by the event.[41]

The American Academy of Pediatrics has stressed the importance of alleviating pain and anxiety for children when they require emergency treatment.[2] A significant portion of the pain children experience when they are in the emergency setting is preventable or can be reduced significantly.[12] A 2010 position statement released by the American College of Emergency Physicians, the Emergency Nurses Association, American Pain Society, and the American Society of Pain Management Nursing states that analgesic management of pain should begin as soon as it is possible if indicated, and should not wait until the pain etiology is determined.[15] Effective management of acute pain and anxiety in children involves an approach that uses both pharmacologic and nonpharmacologic interventions.[12,39,41]

Nonpharmacologic Interventions

Nonpharmacologic pain management begins with decreasing the stress of the child and caregivers throughout the ED visit. Providing a quiet, child-friendly room may begin to alleviate some of the anxieties of being in a noisy rushed ED.[2] Managing stress levels and providing emotional support can decrease anxiety in older children and the perception of the caregivers related to pain in the younger child.[2]

Nonpharmacologic management of pain is used successfully in all ages of children.[12,39,42] For acute pain, it is important to use nonpharmacologic management in addition to medications. The combined outcomes of decreased anxiety and increased coping behaviors result from adequately preparing the child about what to expect before a procedure[42] Engaging the child in decision making promotes their right to be involved in the procedure, to make choices, and to ask questions. This strategy is a positive reinforcement for them that they can help to manage their own pain and anxiety.[42] Allowing the child's caregivers to remain at the bedside during procedures, if possible, may also help to decrease fear and anxiety of the child and caregiver.[12,14,23] The parent or caregiver may need preparation and coaching on how to respond to the child and how to help them cope successfully.[12,23,41] Providing instructions that are clear, and a calm caregiver will increase the probability of successful pain management.[12,41]

Strategies such as age-appropriate distraction, coping statements (I can do this, this will be over soon), guided imagery, and breathing exercises have been used successfully to mitigate pain and stress.[33] Reducing noise or lighting, music, or swaddling may be used with the neonate (refer to **Table 2** for a more comprehensive list of nonpharmacologic techniques for infants and children).[23,35]

Experts believe that play helps to reduce children's anxiety caused by stressful conditions, and regain some control over what they are experiencing.[22] Child life specialist are trained to support children and reduce the impact of stressful or painful experiences, along with preparing them for procedures using medical play.[22,43] In a 2006 paper, the American Academy of Pediatrics stated that "child life services be considered an essential component of quality pediatric healthcare," and that the use of child life is "an indicator of excellence in pediatric care."[22] For those EDs that do not have access to child life services, nonpharmacologic pain management is still possible and a standard best practice. The department should provide training for ED staff on appropriate developmental methods of managing pain and anxiety, and may also create a "distraction toolkit" with books, toys, and electronics such as iPads or games.

Pharmacologic Interventions

For the majority of children, pharmacologic interventions for pain can be safe and therapeutic, although considerations must be made for weight and developmental physiology.[6] There are a number of factors that guide the choice of analgesic therapy for the child presenting to the ED. The pain severity and nature, and the underlying disease or injury may dictate the route and class of medication.[5]

For mild pain, oral medications such as acetaminophen or ibuprofen can be given.[5,44,45] These have opioid-sparing effects and are considered safe; conversely,

Table 2	
Nonpharmacologic therapies for infants and children	
Infants	**Children**
Nonnutritive sucking	Distraction (eg, music, videos, books, toys)
Swaddling	Medical staff coaching
Sucrose	Coping statements
Breast milk[a]	Breathing exercises
Lowered lights	Guided imagery
Music	Positioning
Positioning (eg, facilitated tucking)	Hot or cold therapy
Skin-to-skin contact (15 min before a procedure)	Lighting
Touch or massage	Massage

[a] Breast milk has been found to be developmentally superior to oral sucrose for pain control.[30]
Data from Refs.[5,6,12,39–41]

the use of ibuprofen is controversial in neonates.[22,35,43,44] If the child is ordered to take acetaminophen at home it is important to provide education related to dosing and scheduling. Administering a dose of acetaminophen that is greater than the recommended maximum will increases the risk for hepatic injury.[3,6]

Recommendations for moderate pain are treatment with oral opioids in combination with acetaminophen or ibuprofen.[2,12] Both oral and intranasal routes for opioids are effective and suggested for initial management, if there are not contraindications. The intranasal route has a faster onset and increased bioavailability.[44] Oral codeine, although effective, is poorly metabolized or is hypermetabolized by some patients, so hydrocodone or oxycodone is suggested.[44] Severe pain in children should be treated with intravenous opioids, such as morphine or fentanyl.[6,12] If intravenous access is delayed, the intranasal route may be used.[44] The goal for treatment is to reduce the pain quickly. Administering subtherapeutic doses of medications in multiple doses will only serve to delay relief and increase anxiety, and may exacerbate adverse effects of the analgesic.[12] Single dose opioids may be administered to neonates with the quantity reduced owing to their immature lung, liver, and kidney function.[35] Children should have cardiopulmonary and oxygen monitoring while on opioids, particularly neonates who have an increased risk of apnea.[5,35]

Procedural pain management must consist of appropriate preparation; along with topical and systemic medication, including sedation that is equivalent to the anticipated level of pain. There are many topical anesthetics available for use, some using heat or vibration to optimize their efficacy (**Table 3**).[41] For mild procedural pain in neonates, oral sucrose has been found to be quite effective.[22,39] Nitrous oxide (nitrous) has been widely studied and found to be a safe option for minimal sedation in children.[48,49] Nitrous has analgesic and anxiolytic properties, and has the same efficacy as 10 to 15 mg of morphine when administered at a minimum of 30%.[49]

Table 3
Topical anesthetics

Agent	Use
Eutectic mixture	Intact skin with occlusive dressing 60 min for maximum effect
Lidocaine, prilocaine	Effective for up to 2 h after removal
Liposomal lidocaine	Intact skin with occlusive dressing 30 min for maximum effect
Self-heating lidocaine tetracaine patch	Intact skin 20 min for max effect studied in children ≥3 y
Lidocaine with compressed gas delivery system	Intact skin, max effect within a few minutes
Vapocoolant spray (various anesthetics in the form of a spray)	Spray until slight blanching of skin, works immediately not recommended for those with diminished circulation
Iontophoresis (lidocaine with electric current)	Intact skin maximum effect 10–20 min
Lidocaine/epinephrine/tetracaine (Let)	Apply to open wound maximum effect in 20–30 min. Not for use on mucous membranes
Buzzy	Uses ice and vibration to block pain sensation

Data from Refs.[2,41,46,47]

Use of Pain Protocols

The use of standardized, evidence-based pain protocols or interventions in the ED have been shown to improve pain assessment and management, and patient and caregiver satisfaction.[2,5,41,44] Guidelines, standing orders, or policies should be developed for nurses to administer medications for mild to moderate pain along with topical anesthetics for anticipated procedures, and the use of oral sucrose before procedures for neonates.[2,4,5,44]

SPECIFIC PRESENTATIONS
Abdominal Pain

Some HCP are hesitant to administer analgesics before a diagnosis is made owing to the fears of masking symptoms. A Canadian retrospective review found that only one-half of children with suspected appendicitis received analgesia and almost 25% of those were underdosed.[50] In a survey of emergency physicians who chose not to administer analgesics, 87% were concerned about the surgeon disapproving.[50] Numerous studies support the notion that the administration of analgesics including opioids does not interfere with the diagnosis of appendicitis in children and that they should be treated appropriately for their level of pain.[50–52]

Traumatic Injuries

Musculoskeletal injuries are common in children, and studies have concluded that children do not receive adequate analgesia for fracture pain.[53,54] For uncomplicated arm fractures, Drendel and colleagues[55] conducted a randomized, double-blind trial and found that ibuprofen was as effective as acetaminophen with codeine in managing pain with improved satisfaction of both children and parents. For fracture reduction, a systematic review by Miqita and colleagues[56] revealed that for sedation and analgesia a combination of ketamine and midazolam was superior to fentanyl–midazolam or propofol–fentanyl.

For children who have multisystem trauma, a "multimodal analgesic technique"[56] can be used with a combination of acetaminophen and nonsteroidal antiinflammatory drugs, which may decrease the dosage of opioids required. If opioids are needed, it is suggested to titrate small doses, which will not affect the clinical examination or neurologic assessment.[2] Children may not cope well in the ED after a traumatic accident and will need to have a low-stress, child-friendly atmosphere to decrease anxiety and fear.[56]

Chronic Pain

The most common recurrent or chronic pain in children is headache, followed by abdominal and musculoskeletal pain.[44] Children with chronic conditions that cause pain such as sickle cell disease, osteogenesis imperfecta, cancer, or hemophilia also present to the ED. Pediatric patients with chronic pain may not display the same physical cues or verbalization that patients with acute pain do.[2] This makes the assessment of their pain more difficult.[2,44] The child and their family often have anxiety and fear owing to negative experiences in which the child's pain was not managed well.[44] It is important for the practitioner to use appropriate pain scales and believe the report of the child, even if they are not manifesting physical symptoms. Prompt and appropriate analgesia should be given while "disease-related treatments" are provided.[44] Protocols developed specifically for the disease populations may facilitate treatment and help to decrease variability.[57] In addition, the patient should receive appropriate referrals, because "definitive treatment of chronic pain is not the role of the ED."[58,59]

SUMMARY AND DISCUSSION

It has been well-established that pain management for children in the ED is often inadequate, although there have been improvements owing to medical research and a focus on pediatric pain. As HCP, we have an ethical duty to our patients to provide appropriate pain management. Studies have revealed the importance of adequate pain control for children and there are now many resources available for clinicians related to the topic. Best practice involves use of validated pain scales to evaluate pain, the use of both pharmacologic interventions and child life specialists, and the use of evidence-based protocols to facilitate care.

ACKNOWLEDGMENTS

The author acknowledges L. Patton MSN, RN, PCNS & S. Allen MS, RN, CNS.

REFERENCES

1. The Free Dictionary. Oligoanalgesia. Available at: http://medical-dictionary. thefreedictionary.com/oligoanalgesia. Accessed July 17, 2016.
2. Fein J, Zempsky W, Cravero J, The Committee on Pediatric Emergency Medicine and Section on Anesthesiology and Pain Medicine. Relief of pain and anxiety in pediatric patients in emergency medical systems. Pediatrics 2012;130: e1391–405.
3. Uspai N, Black K, Stephen J. Pediatric pain management in the emergency department. Pediatr Emerg Med Pract 2012;9:1–9. Available at: http://www.ebmedicine. net/topics.php?paction=showTopic&topic_id=348. Accessed August 10.
4. Kleiber C, Jennissen C, MCarthy AM, et al. Evidence-based pediatric pain management in emergency departments of a rural state. J Pain 2011;8:900–10.
5. Bauman B, McManus J. Pediatric pain management in the emergency department. Emerg Med Clin North Am 2005;23:393–414.
6. Baulch I. Assessment and management of pain in the paediatric patient. Nurs Stand 2010;25:35–40.
7. Rafiq A. A brief look at the journey of pain. J Pioneer Med Sci 2013. Available at: http://blogs.jpmsonline.com/2013/05/08/a-brief-look-at-the-journey-of-pain/. Accessed April 20, 2016.
8. Dvorsky G. A brief history of painkillers (and why they work). Daily Explainer 2013. Available at: http://io9.gizmodo.com/how-drugs-work-to-help-you-ease-the-pain-1452216695. Accessed April 20, 2016.
9. Online etymology dictionary. Pain. Available at: http://www.etymonline.com/index. php?term=pain. Accessed July 17, 2016.
10. International Association for the Study of Pain. IASP taxonomy. Available at: http:// www.iasp-pain.org/Taxonomy. Accessed July 13, 2016.
11. McCaffery M. Nursing practice theories related to cognition, bodily pain, and man- environment interactions. Los Angeloc (CA)· University of California at Los Angeles Students' Store; 1968.
12. American Academy of Pediatrics, American Pain Society. The assessment and management of acute pain in infants, children, and adolescents. Pediatrics 2001;108:793–7.
13. American Academy of Pain Medicine. Ethics Charter. 2007. Available at: http:// www.painmed.org/files/ethics-charter.pdf. Accessed July 20, 2016.
14. International Association for the Study of Pain. IASP declaration of Montreal. Statement of access to pain management as a fundamental human right. Available

at: http://www.iasp-pain.org/DeclarationofMontreal?navItemNumber=582.   Accessed June 15, 2016.

15. American College of Emergency Physicians, Emergency Nurses Association, American Pain Society, American Society of Pain Management Nursing. Optimizing the treatment of pain in patients with acute presentations. Policy statement. Ann Emerg Med 2010;56:77–9.

16. Drendel A, Brouseau D, Gorelick M. Pain assessment for pediatric patients in the emergency department. Pediatrics 2006;117:1511–8.

17. Birnie K, Chambers C, Fernandez C, et al. Hospitalized children continue to report undertreated and preventable pain. Pain Res Manag 2014;19:198–204.

18. Clyde C, Kwiatkowski K. Cultural perspective and pain. In: St. Marie B, editor. Core curriculum for pain management nursing. Philadelphia: W.B. Saunders Company; 2002. p. 9–30.

19. Stanford E, Chambers C, Craig K. The role of developmental factors in predicting young children's use of a self-report scale for pain. Pain 2006;120:16–23.

20. Rupp T, Delaney K. Inadequate analgesia in emergency medicine. Ann Emerg Med 2004;43:494–503.

21. Bulloch B, Tenenbein M. Validation of 2 pain scales for use in the pediatric emergency department. Pediatrics 2002;110:1–6.

22. American Academy of Pediatrics Child Life Council and Committee on Hospital Care, Wilson JM. Child life services. Pediatrics 2006;118:1757–63.

23. Srouji R, Rapnapalan S, Schneeweis S. Pain in children: assessment and non-pharmacolgic management. Int J Pediatr 2010;2010:474838.

24. Probst B, Lyons E, Leonard D, et al. Factors affecting emergency department assessment and management of pain in children. J Pediatr Nurs 2005;18:295–9.

25. Johnson CC, Gagnon A, Rennick J, et al. One-on-one coaching to improve pain assessment and management practices of pediatric nurses. J Pediatr Nurs 2007; 22:467–78.

26. Linhares M, Doca F, Martinez F, et al. Pediatric pain: prevalence, assessment, and management in a teaching hospital. Braz J Med Biol Res 2012;45:1287–94.

27. Taylor E, Bovar K, Campbell F. Pain in hospitalized children: a prospective cross-sectional survey of pain prevalence, intensity, assessment, and management in a Canadian pediatric teaching hospital. Pain Res Manag 2008;13:25–32.

28. Stevens B, Abbott L, Yamada J, et al. Epidemiology and management of painful procedures in children in Canadian hospitals. CMAJ 2011;183:e403–10.

29. Herr K, Coyne P, McCaffery M, et al. Pain assessment in the patient unable to self-report: position statement with clinical practice recommendations. Pain Manag Nurs 2011;12:230–50.

30. Pasero C. Pain assessment in infants and young children: premature infant pain profile. Am J Nurs 2002;9:105–6.

31. Merkel S, Voepel-Lewis T, Malviya S. Pain assessment in infants and young children: the FLACC scale. Am J Nurs 2002;102:55–8.

32. O'Rourke D. The measurement of pain in infants, children and adolescents: from policy to practice. Phys Ther 2004;84:560–70.

33. Bulloch B, Garcia-Filion P, Notricia D, et al. Reliability of the color analog scale: repeatability of scores in traumatic and nontraumatic injuries. Acad Emerg Med 2009;16:465–9.

34. Beyer J, Villarruel A, Denyes M. The Oucher user's manual and technical report. 2009. Available at: http://www.oucher.org/downloads/2009_Users_Manual.pdf. Accessed July 31, 2016.

35. Kanwaljeet J. Prevention and treatment of neonatal pain. In: Martin R, Kim M, editors. UpToDate. Waltham (MA): UpToDate. Available at: https://www.uptodate.com/contents/prevention-and-treatment-of-neonatal-pain. Accessed August 1, 2016.

36. Stanford E, Chambers C, Craig K. A normative analysis of the development of pain-related vocabulary in children. Pain 2005;114:278–84.

37. Pasero C, McCaffery M. Pain assessment and pharmacologic management. St Louis (MO): Mosby; 2011.

38. Gallo A. The fifth vital sign: implementation of the neonatal infant pain scale. J Obstet Gynecol Neonatal Nurs 2003;32:199–206.

39. American Academy of Pediatrics. Prevention and management of pain in the neonate: an update. Pediatrics 2006;118:2231–41.

40. Mathews L. Pain in children: unaddressed and mismanaged. Indian J Palliat Care 2011;17:s70–3.

41. Young K. Pediatric procedural pain. Ann Emerg Med 2005;45:161–71.

42. Koller D. Preparing children and adolescents for medical procedures. 2007. Available at: http://www.childlife.org/files/ebppreparationstatement-complete.pdf. Accessed July 30, 2016.

43. Bandstra N, Skinner L, LeBlanc C, et al. The role of child life in pediatric pain management: a survey of child life specialist. J Pain 2008;9:320–9.

44. Krauss B, Calligaris L, Green S. Current concepts in management of pain in children in the emergency department. Lancet 2016;387:83–92.

45. Tsze T, von Baeyer C, Bulloch B, et al. Validation of self-report pain scales in children. Pediatrics 2013;132:e971–9.

46. Hsu G. Topical anesthetics in children. In: Stack A, Wiley J, editors. UptoDate. Waltham (MA): UptoDate. Available at: https://www.uptodate.com/contents/topical-anesthetics-in-children. Accessed August 2, 2016.

47. Buzzy® drug free pain relief. Buzzy website. 2016. Available at: https://buzzyhelps.com/. Accessed August 12, 2016.

48. Babl F, Oakley S, Krieser D. High concentration nitrous oxide for procedural sedation in children: adverse events and depth of sedation. Pediatrics 2008; 121:e528–32.

49. Becker D, Rosenberg M. Nitrous oxide and the inhalation anesthetics. Anesth Prog 2008;55:124–31.

50. Bromberg R, Goldman R. Does analgesia mask diagnosis of appendicitis among children? Cam Fam Physician 2007;53:39–41.

51. Kokki H, Lintula H, Vanamo K, et al. Oxycodone vs placebo in children with undifferentiated abdominal pain: a randomized double blind clinical trial on the effect of analgesia on diagnostic accuracy. Arch Pediatr Adolesc Med 2005;159: 320–5.

52. Kim M, Strait R, Sato T, et al. A randomized clinical trial of analgesia in children with acute abdominal pain. Acad Emorg Med 2002;9:281–7.

53. Brown J, Klein E, Lewis C, et al. Emergency department analgesia for fracture pain. Ann Emerg Med 2003;42:197–205.

54. Kircher J, Drendel A, Newton A, et al. Pediatric musculoskeletal pain in the emergency department: a medical record review of practice variation. CJEM 2014;16: 449–57.

55. Drendel A, Gorelick M, Weisman S, et al. A randomized clinical trial of Ibuprofen versus Acetaminophen with codeine for acute pediatric arm fracture pain. Ann Emerg Med 2009;16:711–6.

56. Miqita R, Klein E, Garrison M. Sedation and analgesia for pediatric fracture reduction I the emergency department: a systematic review. Arch Pediatr Adolesc Med 2006;160:46–51.
57. McFadyen G, Ramaiah R, Bhananker S. Initial assessment and management of pediatric trauma patients. Int J Crit Illn Inj Sci 2012;2(3):121–7.
58. Tanabe P, Myers R, Zosel A, et al. Emergency department management of acute pain episodes in sickle cell disease. Acad Emerg Med 2007;14:419–25.
59. Baker K. Chronic pain syndromes in the emergency department: identifying guidelines for management. Emerg Med Australas 2005;17:57–64.

Unbundling the Bundles

Using Apparent and Systemic Cause Analysis to Prevent Health Care–Associated Infection in Pediatric Intensive Care Units

Terri L. Bogue, MSN, RN, PCNS-BC*, Robert L. Bogue, BS

KEYWORDS

- Health care–associated infections • HAI • Prevention • Apparent cause analysis
- CLABSI • Systemic cause analysis

KEY POINTS

- Prevention of health care–associated infections (HAI) is a priority goal for hospitals and health services.
- Evidence-based prevention bundles reduce the prevalence of HAIs but have not eliminated them.
- The use of apparent cause and systemic cause analysis identify potential causes of HAI.
- Using information from apparent cause and systemic cause analysis provides additional resources to prevent HAI.
- The combination of evidence-based prevention bundles, apparent cause, and systemic cause analysis can significantly reduce HAI rates.

INTRODUCTION

The Centers for Disease Control and Prevention (CDC) estimates there are approximately 1.7 million new cases of health care–associated infections (HAI) every year. Of these cases, approximately 75,000 result in death, making HAIs 1 of the top 10 causes of death in the United States.[1] Not only are these infections implicated in increased morbidity and mortality, they also have significant financial impact on health care facilities through reduced reimbursement, fines, and penalties.

The effects of HAI are clearly evident in the pediatric intensive care unit (PICU) populations, with an HAI prevalence as high as 12%.[2] The effects of these HAIs are demonstrated in increased morbidity, mortality, length of stay, and cost of care.[3]

Disclosure Statement: The authors have nothing to disclose.
Thor Projects LLC, 106 Jordan Court, Carmel, IN 46032, USA
* Corresponding author.
E-mail address: tbogue@thorprojects.com

Among HAIs in the PICU, central line–associated bloodstream infections (CLABSI) are the most commonly reported, followed by ventilator-associated pneumonia (VAP) and catheter-associated urinary tract infections (CA-UTI).[4] The use of invasive devices in this high-risk population, including arterial catheters, central venous catheters, endotracheal tubes, and indwelling urinary catheters, significantly increases the risk of HAI.[3] The patients' normal physical defenses and immunity are compromised because of the severity of their illness requiring intensive care unit level of care in addition to the use of multiple invasive devices increasing their susceptibility.[4]

The hallmark component of an HAI is that the infection is associated with a hospitalization, while a patient is in the hospital for some other cause. In addition to CLABSI, VAP, and CA-UTI, HAIs include surgical site infection (SSI), *Clostridium difficile* (*C diff*), and methicillin-resistant *Staphylococcus aureus*. These infections cause significant harm to patients and increase exposure to antibiotics, which can lead to antibiotic resistance.

The US Department of Health and Human Services has identified reduction of HAIs as an Agency Priority Goal and is committed to demonstrating significant, quantitative, and measurable reductions in HAI.[5] Agency Priority Goals are 2-year single-agency goals that target areas that agency leaders want to improve through focused senior leadership attention. The US government and health care leaders alike have identified the reduction of HAIs as a primary focus to improve patient outcomes.

The Centers for Medicare and Medicaid Services (CMS) have implemented hospital-acquired condition (HAC) programs to incentivize hospitals to reduce HACs, which include CLABSI, CA-UTI, and SSI. These programs impose a 1% reimbursement penalty to the hospitals that rank in the lowest 25% in relation to HAC quality measures.[6] In addition to HAC penalties, CMS has also implemented the hospital value-based purchasing program, which further holds providers accountable for patient outcomes. The value-based purchasing program includes CA-UTI and SSI among other metrics. These penalties will be fully implemented in 2017 with a total of a 2% annual reimbursement withholding.[7] Both of these mandatory programs disrupt the fee-for-service business model for health care facilities.

Evidence-based practices and information related to the prevention of HAIs are well published and recognized. Implementation of appropriate care bundles is a key component to the prevention of HAIs.

The Institute of Healthcare Improvement developed the concept of "bundles" to help health care providers more reliably deliver the best possible care for patients undergoing particular treatments with inherent risks.[8] A "bundle" is an evidence-based process of providing care that typically includes 3 to 5 specific practices that, if performed collectively and reliably, have been proven to improve patient outcomes. However, even when these bundles are performed reliably, patients still develop HAIs. Understanding the potential causes of HAIs has significant impact on preventing future events and keeping patients safe. The Joint Commission requires comprehensive systematic analysis or root cause analysis (RCA) of every sentinel event. A sentinel event is defined as "a patient safety event not primarily related to the natural course of the patient's illness or underlying condition that reaches a patient and results in death, permanent harm, or severe temporary harm."[9] These analyses follow a systematic format and identify basic and causal factors underlying variations in performance that may produce unexpected and undesired adverse outcomes. The outcome of the analysis helps determine process changes that make variations and adverse events less likely to occur in the future. HAIs are not considered sentinel events by the Joint Commission, even though they can lead to death, permanent harm, or more frequently, severe temporary harm. Although an RCA is not required for HAIs by regulatory guidelines, the use of an apparent cause analysis (ACA) of individual events, followed with a systemic cause analysis (SCA) of multiple events, can provide insights into barriers leading to bundle noncompliance, and thereby identify potential opportunities to prevent future HAIs.

The ACA and SCA are 2 of the most important tools available to identify and address system problems, proximate causes, and underlying causes that frequently lead to HAIs. These processes can be completed by consultants or by training staff in the specific techniques. These processes have already demonstrated rapid improvement in several facilities. The information gained in a specific facility is likely to lead to improvements that are generalizable to other organizations.

When reviewing HAIs, an ACA provides different views and information and supports the identification of multiple variations that may impact the patient and be associated with HAIs. The ACA also provides the opportunity to find multiple specific solutions to prevent future infections with the same or similar causes. An SCA is the in-depth review of a series of infections to discover trends or more opportunities for widespread improvements. The SCA reviews multiple infections and finds common trends that may be impacting a greater number of patients. The SCA provides a broader view to change practices as necessary based on trends rather than individual events and leads to hospital-wide improvement in patient outcomes. The ACA is similar to looking at the proverbial iceberg (**Fig. 1**) and includes the obvious iceberg and some of the hidden factors, whereas the SCA uncovers the hidden factors and trends that lead to multiple HAIs.

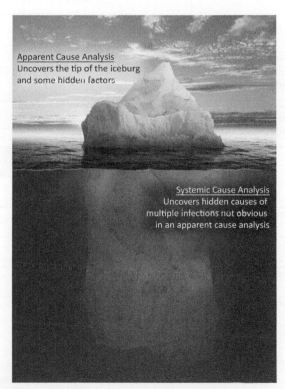

Apparent Cause Analysis
Uncovers the tip of the iceburg and some hidden factors

Systemic Cause Analysis
Uncovers hidden causes of multiple infections not obvious in an apparent cause analysis

Fig. 1. ACA/SCA iceberg analogy.

APPARENT CAUSE ANALYSIS

The ACA helps to identify the obvious and the not-so-obvious causes of individual HAI events. The ACA commonly takes several hours to initiate and frequently requires several days to complete. The conclusion of the ACA reveals the story of the patient and uncovers most of the contributing factors that influenced the HAI event. The steps of an ACA need to be standardized and conscientiously followed to ensure that each HAI is reviewed consistently and completely. The use of a standard template (**Figs. 2–4**) ensures the same information is evaluated each time an ACA is completed, thus improving the effectiveness of the process.

The use of a standardized template for the ACA also provides data to be used in the future SCA process. The steps of the ACA are noted in **Fig. 5**; following these systematic steps supports a consistent review of HAI events.

If not completed in a manner designed to support staff and build trust, an ACA can feel like a witch hunt: looking for someone to blame for harming a patient. An ACA can only be effective when it is completed in a nonjudgmental manner without assigning personal blame and while also supporting the staff. All staff have to have a high confidence that the ACA is completed to help keep patients safe through improvements,

[a]Date of infection				
[a]Unit				
Name				
[a]MRN				
Admit Date [a]LOS				
DOB [a]Age and Weight				
Diagnosis				
[a]Organism (s):				
Results and location of all culture(s) within 72 h of infection				
[a]Travel/procedure in 96 h prior to positive culture				
[a]Isolation (Yes/No)				
	Day of infection	24 h prior	48 h prior	72 h prior
Blood products (Yes/No)				
Temperature range				
WBC count				
[a]CHG bath and daily linen change				
[a]Patient Hand Hygiene				
[a]Appropriate oral care				

Fig. 2. ACA CLABSI template patient information. [a] Indicates information used for SCA. CHG, chlorhexidine gluconate; DOB, date of birth; LOS, length of stay; MRN, medical record number; WBC, white blood cell.

Patient name				
[a] Infected line type If PICC: sutured or stat locked?				
Date/ location/ provider who inserted infected line				
[a] Age of infected line				

Location of other active lines during 72
  h prior to infection and dates
  placed				

[a]Dressing changes Date/reason				
[a]Cap changes Date/reason				
[a]Tubing changes Date/reason				
Florastor/Floranex/Culturelle Pediatric specific				
	Day of Infection	24 h prior	48 h prior	72 h prior
Line use				
[a]TPN (Yes/No)				
[a]Line complications (daily flush/draw)				
IVP medications Number to assess #of access				
# of heparin flushes				
# Lab draw				
[a]Total number of IVP/labs/heparin (assume 2 accesses with each access for waste/flush)				
[a]TPA or Ethanol				

Fig. 3. ACA CLABSI template device information. [a] Indicates information used for SCA. IVP, intravenous piggy back; PICC, peripherally inserted central catheter; TPA, tissue plasminogen activator; TPN, total parenteral nutrition.

and that punitive actions are never the outcome of an ACA, but rather that they are a learning opportunity. It can take time and experience to build this culture of trust in an organization if it does not currently exist. The culture of safety that develops into trust requires the creation of an open, free, nonpunitive environment in which health care professionals can feel safe to report adverse events.[10] If this is not done consistently, the value of information obtained and the ability of the ACA and SCA to implement change are greatly hampered.

Like an RCA, the ACA searches for 3 basic types of causes: physical causes, human causes, and organizational causes.[9] Physical causes include the failure of equipment or tangible items; this may include central line catheters, caps, or dressings.

Human causes include personnel doing something incorrectly or omitting a procedure required item, such as hand hygiene or not scrubbing the catheter hub. When looking at human failure, like all failure, it is important to look for the "why." That is, why was

Patient name	
RN Day of infection 24 h prior: Night 24 h prior: Day 48 h prior: Night 48 h prior: Day 72 h prior: Night 72 h prior: Day Physician Resident Nurse Practitioner Clinical Nurse Specialist Pharm D PT/OT PCA	
Comments from Infection Prevention	
Misc. information	
Recommendations [a]Huddle results	
Plan for implementation of new information	

Fig. 4. ACA CLABSI template device results. [a] Indicates information used for SCA. PCA, patient care associate; PT/OT, physical therapist/occupational therapist; RN, registered nurse.

something not done? Taiichi Ohno, the chief architect of the Toyota Production System, included the 5-whys questioning process to be used when attempting to unravel the causes of problems and spark ideas for innovative solutions.[11] This process requires the analyst to ask "why" to a question at least 5 times to get to the heart of the causal chain of a problem.

It is imperative to continue asking why when completing an ACA, rather than accepting the obvious and easy answer. This obvious or easy answer will frequently not identify the underlying cause of the event and does not take into account the complexity of health care, therefore missing vital information necessary to prevent future infections. When determining human causes, it is necessary to consider the cause for the failure, not simply assigning blame. The underlying cause that resulted in the human failure will lead to a solution that has long-term impact and will support the staff in participating in future ACAs by building trust.

The final type of cause to review is organizational causes. These organizational causes include policies, procedure information, or other organizational processes that are flawed in some way. Frequently, there is not one apparent cause of an event, even though there may be a cause found early in the ACA process that seems to identify the problem. If one continues looking beyond the obvious, there are frequently a series of events that lead to an infection. The Swiss cheese model (**Fig. 6**) is the description patient safety experts use to demonstrate how a combination of events aligns in a manner that results in harm. The layers of protection are

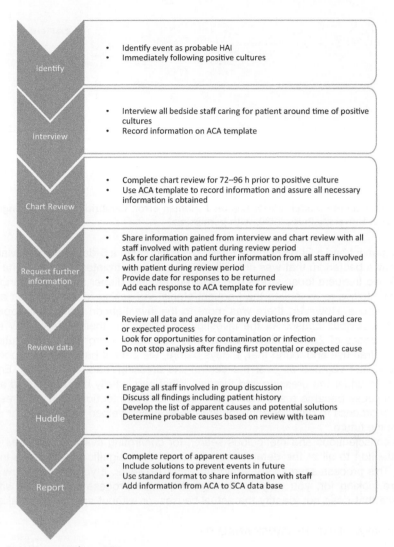

Fig. 5. Steps to complete ACA.

like slices of Swiss cheese, incidents and variations in practice align in the perfect order to make it through the series of holes in the Swiss cheese slices and result in patient harm. In many cases, there are a series of events or practices that do not follow standard practices that align in just the precise manner that the results are harm to a patient.

One of the most important aspects of performing the ACA is to keep an open mind and continue to look for different possibilities, rather than accept the first or most obvious cause. Daniel Kahneman,[12] in *Thinking Fast and Slow*, discusses the impact of confirmation bias, the work of Peter Wason,[13] and the natural tendency to believe the initial construction of the best possible interpretation of a situation as confirmation bias. The initial belief developed by the analyst is based on operations of the associative memory and can lead the analyst of an ACA to results that are not accurate. In one

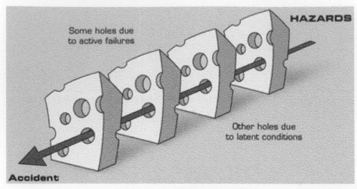

Fig. 6. Swiss cheese model. (*From* Reason J. Human error. Cambridge (United Kingdom): Cambridge: University Press; 1990; with permission.)

case, a patient had a CLABSI in the PICU. The patient had a 5-day-old subclavian line and grew a bacterium that was normally found in the gastrointestinal tract. The child was having frequent loose stools that required frequent diaper and linen changes. It seemed intuitive to associate the frequent stools and soiling to the infection as the obvious cause. However, there was more to the investigation than what appeared to be the obvious cause. As the investigators continued their review, they found frequent doses of Zofran administered. They continued searching for the rationale for the Zofran use and found that, 2 days before, the patient had positive blood cultures and had vomited all over the central line dressing, cap, and tubing. Emesis had gotten under the dressing and the cap. What had initially been identified as the obvious cause became a secondary risk factor for this infection. This ACA resulted in a new process to care for contaminated lines, which helped reduce similar infections in the future.

The conscientious and meticulous search for confirming evidence requires effort and attention to all of the details, regardless of how insignificant they may initially seem. This process seems very straightforward. However, if you do not know what you are looking for, you may go through the entire process of an ACA with an outcome that does not identify the actual causes, or without any outcome at all.

CASE REVIEW APPARENT CAUSE ANALYSIS
Identify

A 9-year-old patient, G.G., in the PICU developed positive blood cultures growing *Klebsiella pneumoniae* from a 45-day-old tunneled central venous catheter. It is important to note, *K pneumoniae* is normally found in human intestines and feces. According to the CDC, in health care settings, *K pneumoniae* can be spread through person-to-person contact or by contamination of the environment.[14] This infection occurred more than 2 days after the patient was admitted to the hospital, ruling out the potential for the infection to be considered present on admission. Recognizing the length of time that the line was in place supports the conclusion of a maintenance issue, not an insertion-related infection, as insertion-related infections develop within 72 to 96 hours after insertion of device.

Interview

Interviews were completed with bedside nursing staff, physicians, and therapist; each reported appropriate hand hygiene and clean gloves as well as isolation precautions for long-term contact isolation. There were reports of the patient having frequent large stools, frequently itching in their diaper, and the patient refusing to wash their hands. No one remembers any issues with the central line flushing or being unable to get a blood return from the line.

Chart Review

The review of the chart revealed 4 sets of blood cultures, all of which grew *K pneumoniae*. No complications related to the central line were documented, although the dressing was changed before due for undocumented causes; tubing and cap changes were completed and documented when due. The patient had frequent diarrhea; linen changes were completed more frequently than expected. The central line was accessed 9 to 11 times per day. However, a heparin flush was not provided after each access even though fluids were not infusing. The patient had a daily chlorhexidine gluconate bath and linen change per hospital policy. Neither ethanol locks nor alteplase was used to treat problems with the central line, and no blood products were infused during the 72 hours before positive cultures.

Request for Further Information

Review of case to date was shared with staff (**Box 1**), ideally via e-mail, to all staff who provided care for the patient during the 72 to 96 hours before the event date. Further information was requested related to patient and staff related to hand hygiene, use of gloves when required, bundle compliance, use and function of line, integrity of central line and dressing, and any concerns or potential risks.

Review Data

Data from interviews, the chart review, and responses to the ACA request for information were reviewed. New information obtained from request for further information revealed that the early dressing change was completed because of nonocclusion. G.G. frequently scratched everywhere, including inside her diaper, around her central line, and the central line dressing; she refused to have her hands washed. Frequently, diarrhea was large enough to leak into the bed, requiring more frequent linen changes.

Huddle

The team is brought together and discusses the findings to date. The most probable cause was the patient contaminating her central line dressing and site with bacteria from her fingernails and hands after scratching in her pants followed by scratching her central line dressing and surrounding area. Large diarrhea was not always able to be cleaned before the patient could get her hands in it. G.G.'s hands were wiped clean when visibly soiled; however, her nails were not trimmed or cleaned. Following the huddle, a plan was developed for this patient that included scheduled hand hygiene for the patient, including a sign customized with the patient's favorite cartoon character (ie, Doc McStuffins) to post in the patient's room to remind patient, visitors, and staff to wash their hands at the appropriate times.

Report

A standardized report is developed based on the findings of the ACA. This information is placed in an easy-to-review template that outlines risks involved in the event, and any new practices that are being implemented to reduce future risk. A plan for necessary education or interventions is developed and implemented. The standardized report (**Fig. 7**) from the ACA is shared with all staff house-wide. Sharing this information without blame allows more effective diffusion of the knowledge that is

---

Box 1
Apparent cause analysis request for information

On 6/21/2016, G.G. was diagnosed with a CLABSI; *K pneumoniae* grew in blood cultures drawn from her 45-day-old tunneled central line.

K pneumoniae is normally found in the human mouth, skin, and intestines. In health care settings, *K pneumoniae* can be spread through person-to-person contact.

In an effort to understand what may have been occurring with this patient and to heighten awareness about the importance of meticulous central line care, each of the health care providers assigned to care for G.G. during the 72 hours before the positive cultures is receiving this request. Please review the information and share your insight to assist in determining apparent causes for this CLABSI.
- I want to share with you what I gathered from the patient's chart related to possible infection risk.
- Four sets of blood cultures were drawn on 6/21 after a temperature of 39.0°C; all grew *K pneumoniae*.
- No complications with the line are documented.
- There was one dressing change on 6/19; this was 2 days before a routine dressing change was due. It is unknown why the dressing was changed.
- It was not documented that the line was flushed and clamped when not in use.
- Daily bath and linen change were documented.
- Tubing and cap changes were documented per policy.
- G.G. had frequent diarrhea.
- It is reported that G.G. frequently itched in her pants.
- It is reported that G.G. refused to have her hands washed.

As you are thinking about the information you can share with me, please consider:
- Was hand hygiene completed and clean gloves donned before any manipulation of the line?
- Was a complete 15-second scrub and 15-second dry used for all access?
- Was appropriate hand hygiene completed?
- Were high touch surfaces wiped each shift?
- Were there any breaches in technique, processes, integrity of the line or dressings?
- Was the line flushed and clamped after each use?
- Was there anything occurring with the patient that you would consider a risk?
- Did you have any concerns that you want to share?

The information you share will not only help determine the possible causes of this infection, but, more importantly, it can also help us identify opportunities to keep our patients safer in the future.

Please include any information you remember; if you have nothing that seems important, please let me know that as well.

It is very important to have your response by 6/25/2016. You are also requested to attend a huddle to discuss this infection and ways to prevent future infections. Your input is necessary to develop better methods of preventing CLABSI.

---

necessary for change. This process of diffusing knowledge is outlined in *Diffusion of Innovation* as part of the diffusion process through which an innovation is communicated through certain channels over time among the members of a social system.[15] The process of innovation-decision outlines the thought patterns and processes through which an individual passes from the point of obtaining new knowledge, developing an attitude about the new knowledge, deciding to adopt the new practice or not, and finally, to implementation and use of the new information consistently in practice.[15] The diffusion process must be considered as new ideas in infection prevention, based on the information from an ACA that is disseminated.

CLABSI Huddle results:

18th CLABSI in 2016
Patients: GG[a]
Age: 9 y old
Unit: Ped

- Positive blood cultures: Klebsiella pneumoniae x4
- Klebsiella pneumoniae typically found in intestine and feces
- 45 d old tunneled central line

The risks identified that can lead to harm:

RISK FACTORS

- Frequent diarrhea
- Central line dressing found non-occlusive
- Pt scratching in diaper
- Pt scratching central line dressing and surrounding area
- Pt refused hand hygiene

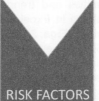

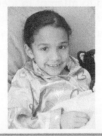

Individual missed opportunities

- Patient nails not clipped and cleaned routinely
- Hand hygiene allowed to be refused by patient

Hand hygiene plan
- **Wash hands**
  - **Before and after eating and oral meds**
  - **After going to bathroom or diaper change**
  - **When needed due to soiling**
- **Nails clipped weekly**
- **Nails cleaned daily and as needed**

Terri Bogue MSN, RN, PCNS –BC

Fig. 7. ACA report ([a] indicates that this in not a real patient). (© 2016 AvailTek LLC.)

At the completion of each ACA cycle, pertinent information from the ACA is entered into a database to compare the findings of this event with those of previous and future events. The conclusion of the ACA process begins the SCA process.

SYSTEMIC CAUSE ANALYSIS

The SCA is the systematic analysis and evaluation of a collection of seemingly disparate past events to identify similarities in causes among a larger group of infections.

The SCA is comparable to looking at the underwater portion of an iceberg and finding information that was previously invisible. The apparent causes of individual infections can identify a wide variety of potential barriers and areas requiring improvement within a health care system. When completing an SCA, it is important to identify the primary and secondary apparent causes from all HAI types using data from completed ACA. A standardized method is necessary to compare data from completed ACAs for similarities and trends. One method to facilitate on-going SCAs is to develop a database in Excel that allows for multiple search options. The data noted with an asterisk in **Figs. 2–4** provide the outline for a database to evaluate all events through the SCA process. Once a method of evaluation is determined, data from each ACA are added after each event, and further SCAs are completed using the new information. The various infections are compared for any similarities that may be included: causal organism, patient unit, as well as any other data that may lead to new insight or information (**Fig. 8**). This evaluation identifies common causes across various HAIs that can lead to new prevention strategies. Typically, an SCA is completed monthly or quarterly depending on the number of events that occur. At least 3 events are preferred to complete an SCA to be able to identify new opportunities. After a spike in HAI, an SCA should be completed to attempt to identify any underlying causes. When looking closely at the entire group of infections and comparing details, you may find a problem you never knew existed—one with overwhelming consequences.

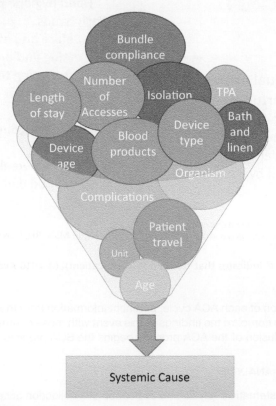

Fig. 8. SCA process.

CASE STUDY SYSTEMIC CAUSE ANALYSIS

A specific unit in the hospital was having a significant spike in their CLABSIs. ACAs had been completed after each CLABSI; they identified a variety of potential causes ranging from hand hygiene to contaminated central lines. As the SCA was being completed, it became apparent that the spike in CLABSI correlated directly with the implementation of a new closed blood draw system on that unit. The infections began occurring within 6 weeks after the new system was implemented. This new system allowed blood to be drawn from a central line without requiring a waste. The same lumen could also be used for infusions between blood draws. This device was difficult to clear blood from, the blood remaining in the device combined with infusing total parenteral nutrition proving to be a perfect breeding ground for bacteria. The new device was also more difficult to use and appeared to be requiring more manipulation, which could lead to further possible contamination. After recognizing this factor, the investigators started reviewing all the cases again to determine if the device in question was being used on these patients. It was soon evident that many of the infections during the last 2 months occurred in patients wherein the new device was being used. There had been a 300% increase in CLABSI during a 3-month period on this specific unit. ACAs had been completed following each CLABSI; each one found something a little different from previous infections. It was not until the infections were reviewed together that the systemic cause was identified and effective steps were taken to reduce risk. The new device was removed from the hospital, and the CLABSI rate rapidly returned to its predevice state.

As new products are used, it is important to note any changes in incidents or infections that may occur. A formal process must be used to assure unintended outcomes do not occur.

RESULTS

The prevention of HAIs can be complicated and at times can feel overwhelming. The effective utilization of appropriate evidence-based bundles is proven to reduce HAI. Maintaining bundle compliance greater than 95%, which is necessary for maximal impact, is difficult. Adding the effective use of the ACA and SCA process adds awareness and identifies opportunities for additional steps to prevent HAI in a facility. In the pediatric hospital where these 2 processes were used systematically as a key intervention, there was a 14% house-wide reduction in CLABSI in a single year. During this time, bundle compliance varied between 62% and 82% with a mean of 73%. The impact of the effective use of the ACA and SCA process cannot be minimized.

SUMMARY

Health care today requires quality care for all patients; preventing HAIs is a key component of quality care. The prevention of these infections is a national goal and important to patients and health care facilities around the globe. The financial impact of reducing HAI is significant because it directly reduces hospital cost.

The implementation of bundles to guide care and prevent HAIs is well documented. The relationship between bundle compliance and HAI prevention is a direct correlation, with a sustained compliance of greater than 95% required for maximal improvement.[16] Although the importance of bundle compliance cannot be underestimated, ACA and SCA are additional tools that help achieve HAI goals. The use of ACA and SCA is an effective method to systematically identify potential causes and HAIs and discover opportunities to prevent future infections. It is necessary to follow a systematic process for these analyses to be most effective. The importance of a systematic process to identify probable causes cannot be minimized, whereas a culture of trust among staff is essential in obtaining accurate information. The effectiveness of the ACA and SCA is dependent on reliable information and the participation of all health care providers. With reliable information and effective ACA and SCA processes, interventions can be implemented that will prevent future infections.

It is necessary to follow a standardized process to complete an ACA after every HAI event. The ACAs must then be followed with SCAs comparing data from similar and dissimilar events. The SCA supports the discovery of common causes of multiple infections that are frequently missed in an ACA. These "common causes" have the potential to affect multiple patients and cause many infections that do not appear to be related when viewed individually. The benefit of the SCA can be significantly greater than the benefit of any single ACA. However, without the individual ACA, the necessary information for the SCA would not be available.

Although the process of reviewing every HAI is not required by regulatory bodies, the use of ACA and SCA is extremely effective in finding opportunities to prevent HAIs. These processes can identify facility-specific issues and uncover yet-to-be-discovered barriers that may affect patients in multiple facilities. Learning to complete ACAs and SCAs takes time and practice, but the life you save may change the world.

REFERENCES

1. Centers for Disease Control and Prevention. Identifying Healthcare-associated Infections for NHSN Surveillance. 2016. Available at: http://www.cdc.gov/nhsn/pdfs/pscmanual/pcsmanual_current.pdf. Accessed July 1, 2016.
2. Smulders CA, van Gestel JP, Bos AP. Are central line bundles and ventilator bundles effective in critically ill neonates and children. Intensive Care Med 2013;39:1352–8.
3. Nowak JE, Brilli RJ, Lake MR, et al. Reducing catheter-associated bloodstream infections in the pediatric intensive care unit: business case for quality improvement. Pediatr Crit Care Med 2010;11(5):579–87.
4. Northway T, Langley JM, Skippen P. Healthcare-associated infection in the pediatric intensive care unit. In: Fulman JJ, Zimmerman BP, editors. Pediatric critical care. 4th edition. Philadelphia: Mosby; 2011. p. 1506–19.
5. Office of Disease Prevention and Health Promotion. National Action Plan to Prevent Health Care Associated Infections. 2016. Available at: http://health.gov/hcq/prevent-hai.asp. Accessed July 1, 2016.
6. Quality Net. Hospital-Acquired Condition (HAC) Reduction Program. 2016. Available at: https://www.qualitynet.org/dcs/ContentServer?c=Page&pagename=QnetPublic%2FPage%2FQnetTier2&cid=1228774189166. Accessed July 5, 2016.
7. Quality Net. Hospital value-based purchasing overview. 2016. Available at: https://www.qualitynet.org/dcs/ContentServer?c=Page&pagename=QnetPublic%2FPage%2FQnetTier2&cid=1228772039937. Accessed July 5, 2016.
8. Haraden C. Improvement stories, what is a bundle? Institute for Healthcare Improvement. 2016. Available at: http://www.ihi.org/resources/Pages/ImprovementStories/WhatIsaBundle.aspx. Accessed July 1, 2016.
9. Joint Commission. Root cause analysis in health care: tools and techniques. 5th edition. Oak Brook (IL): Joint commission Resources; 2015.
10. Weick KE, Sutcliffe KM. Managing the unexpected: resilient performance in an age of uncertainty. 2nd edition. San Francisco (CA): Jossey-Bass; 2007.

11. Christensen CM, Dyer J, Gregersen H. The innovator's DNA: mastering the five skills of disruptive innovators. Boston: Harvard Business Review Press; 1994.
12. Kahneman D. Thinking fast and slow. New York: Farrar, Straus and Giroux; 2011.
13. Wason PC. On the failure to eliminate hypotheses in a conceptual task. Q J Exp Psychol 1960;12(3):129–40.
14. Centers for Disease Control and Prevention. Klebsiella pneumoniae in Healthcare Settings. 2016. http://www.cdc.gov/HAI/organisms/klebsiella/klebsiella.html. Accessed July 1, 2016.
15. Rogers EM. Diffuison of innovation. 5th edition. New York: Simon & Schurster; 2003.
16. Furuya EY, Dick A, Perencevich EN, et al. Central line bundle implementation in US intensive care units and impact on bloodstream infections. PLoS One 2011; 6(1):e15452.

Putting the Family Back in the Center

A Teach-Back Protocol to Improve Communication During Rounds in a Pediatric Intensive Care Unit

Terri L. Bogue, MSN, RN, PCNS-BC[a],*, Lynn Mohr, PhD, APN, PCNS-BC, CPN[b]

KEYWORDS

- Patient and family–centered care • PFCC • Interdisciplinary rounds • PICU
- Teach-back • Patient-centered care • Pediatric

KEY POINTS

- Patients and their families relate effective communication with quality of care.
- Inclusion of patients and families in interdisciplinary rounds is a component of patient and family–centered care.
- Ensuring that patients and families understand what is discussed during interdisciplinary rounds is necessary to support patient and family–centered care.
- Implementation of a protocol that includes explanation of rounds, prerounding and postrounding, and shared patient care plan for the day to increase the family's satisfaction and patient outcomes.
- The use of the teach-back method ensures that the family understands the discussions completed during interprofessional rounds and the plan of care for the child.

BACKGROUND

Patient and family–centered care (PFCC), also known as patient-centered care, is recognized as an innovative approach to the planning, delivery, and evaluation of health care. PFCC is grounded in a mutually beneficial partnership among patients, families, and health care providers that recognizes the importance of the family in the patient's life. Inclusion of the patient's primary caregiver in daily bedside rounds with the entire interdisciplinary team is a current standard of PFCC.

Disclosure: Funding and education sessions for this project were supplied through a grant from American Association of Critical Care Nurses as part of the Clinical Scene Investigator program.
[a] Thor Projects LLC, 106 Jordan Court, Carmel, IN 46032, USA; [b] Pediatric & Neonatal CNS Programs, College of Nursing, Rush University, 606 South Paulina Suite 1080N, Chicago, IL 60612, USA
* Corresponding author.
E-mail address: tbogue@thorprojects.com

Crit Care Nurs Clin N Am 29 (2017) 233–250
http://dx.doi.org/10.1016/j.cnc.2017.01.009
0899-5885/17/© 2017 Elsevier Inc. All rights reserved.

ccnursing.theclinics.com

Preparation of the family before interdisciplinary rounds, followed by validation of comprehension of the discussion related to the child and the plan of care after rounds, is extremely valuable, but none of these are frequently provided or even considered. In the pediatric intensive care unit (PICU), the complexity of care, critical condition of the patient, the stress of having a critically ill child, and minimal levels of health literacy make this preparation even more vital.

In the PICU, interdisciplinary rounds are frequently completed outside the patient's room each morning. The interdisciplinary team (consisting of the intensivist, bedside nurse, nurse practitioner, residents, fellow, pharmacist, and respiratory therapist; consulting groups, social workers, and dieticians may also join in daily rounds as required by the patient's condition) gathers to discuss the patient's condition and plan of care. The patient's family is frequently invited to participate with the interdisciplinary team in rounds each day. The process for rounding is fairly standardized: the resident presents a brief history of the patient's condition; conducts a review of medications, laboratory findings, and current problems; and discusses any issues that occurred overnight or in the morning before rounds. When the resident completes the overview of the patients' status, the bedside nurse adds or clarifies any information, and relays any nursing or family concerns. Following the nurse's overview of the patient and discussion of the family's concerns, the respiratory therapist discusses any respiratory treatments or inhaled medications the patient is receiving, and reviews the patient's response to these therapies. After the patient overview is presented, a systematic plan is formulated, orders are written, and then resident education related to disease process or unusual changes is completed by the attending physician, and at that point any unanswered questions from the family or the team are answered. The family is encouraged to participate in rounds as members of their child's interdisciplinary care team. However, in this environment, many family members are uncomfortable revealing their lack of understanding of complicated medical terms. They do not want to interrupt the physician or appear unknowledgeable. Thus, family members' questions may go unanswered because of a lack of understanding or not being asked, or they may misunderstand the plan of care for their child.[1]

The scope of the problem is evident through the use of questionnaires mailed to families after discharge from the hospital. Data gleaned from these questionnaires show that caregivers do not understand what was told to them, and that they do not think they had enough input or say in their child's care (**Fig. 1**).

PFCC supports the inclusion of family as important partners in health care. Enabling family members to fulfill this role in an effective manner requires that they understand their child's condition and the proposed plan of care. A change in current practice is required to support the family's understanding and ability to actively participate in improving their child's care. This article discusses an evidence-based protocol that was developed to improve families' participation and understanding of their children's conditions and plans of care.

LITERATURE REVIEW

PFCC is considered the standard of care in many clinical practice settings and has been widely endorsed by multiple organizations. The Institute of Medicine (IOM), 2001[2]; American College of Critical Care Medicine (ACCM), 2007[1]; and the American Academy of Pediatrics (AAP), 2012[3]; have publicly endorsed PFCC. The recommendations embedded within these endorsements include several defined responsibilities that outline specific expectations for current practice. The 2001 IOM report, *Crossing the Quality Chasm*, made specific recommendations for changes to the health care

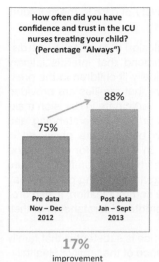
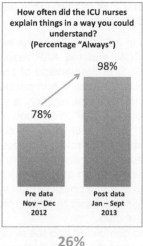
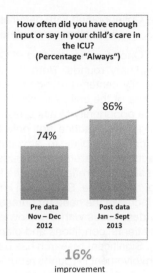

Fig. 1. Patient/family satisfaction data. (*Data from* National Research Corporation, Lincoln, NE.)

system.[2] These recommendations emphasize the need for PFCC and the ongoing and open exchange of information between health care providers and patients.[2] The IOM further defines PFCC as care that is respectful of and responsive to individual patient preferences, needs, and values.[1] Research further shows that the primary need of patients and families is the need for information.[4] Patients and families need answers that are accurate and presented in a way that is understandable. Common to all such interactions is the desire for trustworthy information that is attentive, responsive, and tailored to an individual's needs.[2]

The ACCM strongly endorsed PFCC specifically as defined by the IOM in 2001. The IOM report further stressed that patient and family involvement can profoundly influence clinical decisions and patient outcomes in intensive care units (ICUs).[1] The ACCM supports this care model because of its recognition that critically ill patients are frequently unable to fully participate in their own health care decisions. If families are not included in the decision making and daily care of their loved ones, they are unprepared and feel less supported when they are asked to make decisions related to their loved ones' care.[1]

PFCC recognizes the vital role that families play in ensuring the health and well-being of children and family members of all ages. The AAP guidelines (2012) provide 5 principles that form the foundation of the pediatrician's role related to PFCC. These principles include:

Listening to and respecting individual children and their families
Ensuring flexibility in policies, procedures, and practices to tailor care to fulfill the specific needs, beliefs, and cultural values of individual children and their families while facilitating appropriate choices related to approaches to care
Consistently sharing complete, honest, and unbiased information with patients and their families in useful and meaningful ways to promote effective participation in care and decision making
Providing formal and informal support for each child and family during each phase of the child's life

Collaborating with patients and their families in the delivery of care to the individual child in all aspects of health care[3]

One step in providing PFCC in a PICU involves the inclusion of families in interdisciplinary rounds. Both the ACCM and the AAP recommend that interdisciplinary family-centered rounds take place at the bedside of critically ill children in the presence of the child's family.[1] During rounds, it is imperative that families are provided the opportunity to ask questions, clarify information, and participate in decision making. This practice not only benefits families through improved understanding and increased ability to advocate for their children, it also benefits the physician in educating parents and residents. This practice provides an example for parents and residents to reflect on in the future, promoting improved communication for the future of health care. Successful implementation of PFCC during the rounding process may decrease the need for nurses to mediate physician-family communication; it also provides nurses with the knowledge and basis to further promote understanding of their patients' conditions and plans of care.[1]

Significant research has been completed and the evidence is substantial that family involvement in rounds requires more than just the attendance of the family.[5] Health literacy, feelings of inclusion and acceptance, and the willingness of the team to remain available to ensure all questions are answered, followed by the development of an inclusive plan of care, are also necessary to successfully fulfill the requirements of PFCC during rounds. A literature matrix was created to support this project (Table 1).

Evidence shows that parents of children in the PICU place great importance on receiving information about their children's conditions, having their questions answered, and talking with the physicians in charge of their children's care.[4] Several studies have shown that the most pressing needs of families of patients in the ICU are the need for information and communication.[6] Parents of children in the PICU view the provision of information and communication with the care team as key components of quality care. Ineffective communication between the health care team and the patient or the patient's family has been identified as a key factor resulting in patient-family dissatisfaction, increased length of stay, and increased negative outcomes.[7]

Comprehensive, state-of-the-art care of patients in the ICU requires not only excellent medical treatment and nursing care but also optimal communication and adequate interaction with the health care team. Consistent communication between the patient/family and the health care team is aided by incorporation of the family in daily interdisciplinary ICU rounds. Evidence shows that inclusion in rounds is important; however, it also shows that failure to comprehend a diagnosis, prognosis, or treatment occurs for 35% to 50% of family members.[5] This finding further supports the need to ensure that families understand the key points of discussion in interdisciplinary rounds. It is not sufficient that families are merely present during interdisciplinary rounds.

Family presence at interdisciplinary rounds promotes the flow of information among all members of the health care team, including the family, and also promotes timely bidirectional communication. This practice supports PFCC and improves outcomes for patients and satisfaction for their families.

THEORETIC FRAMEWORK

The evidence-based practice model was developed by Rosswurm and Larrabee[8] from theoretic and research literature related to evidence-based practice and change theory. This nursing theory guides practitioners through the process of changing to

Table 1
Literature matrix

Citation	Problem Under Study	Participants	Findings	Conclusion
AAP, Committee on Hospital Care and Institute for Patient- and Family-Centered Care, 2012	Development of recommendations for high-quality, FFCC for implementation in pediatrics	NA	PFCC can improve patient and family outcomes, improve the patient's and family's experience, increase patient and family satisfaction, build on child and family strengths, increase professional satisfaction, decrease health care costs, and lead to more effective use of health care resources	Specific recommendations for how pediatricians can integrate PFCC in hospitals, clinics, and community settings, and in broader systems of care
Davison et al, 2007	Develop clinical practice guidelines for the support of the patient and family in the adult, pediatric, or neonatal patient-centered ICU	Multidisciplinary task force of experts in critical care practice from the ACCM and the Society of Critical Care Medicine	Recommendations completed that endorse shared decision making, early and repeated care conferences, honoring culturally appropriate requests, spiritual support, staff education, debriefing to minimize impact of family interactions on staff, family presence at rounds and resuscitation, open flexible visiting hours, and family support	Clinicians must acknowledge the important role that family members and other health care surrogates play in patient care, and embrace their participation
Eggly & Meert, 2011	Parental inclusion in PICU rounds: how does it fit with PFCC?	Parents with children in PICU	Most parents of hospitalized children prefer to be present during rounds and are willing to accept the potential risk of discomfort and lack of privacy. Parents who were present during rounds report having had the opportunity to ask questions, provide information, and participate in decisions, and report feeling better informed and more satisfied	Exploring the perspective of health care professionals and families is a critical step in the careful development and implementation of new programs

(continued on next page)

Table 1
(continued)

Citation	Problem Under Study	Participants	Findings	Conclusion
IOM, 2001	Performance expectations for the twenty-first century health care system	NA	Performance expectations for the twenty-first century health care system, 10 new rules to guide patient-clinician relationships, a framework to better align incentives inherent in payment and accountability with improvement in quality, and key steps to promote evidence-based practice and strengthen clinical information systems	Documents the causes of the quality gap, identifies current practices that impede quality care, and explores how systems approaches can be used to implement change
Kleiber et al,[4] 2006	Families place great importance on receiving information about their child's condition, having their questions answered, and talking with the physician in charge of their child's care	Patients, families, and staff of a 12-bed PICU at Children's Hospital of Iowa	Opening the PICU to patients' families during bedside round has beneficial effects for parents, children, and the health care team	Parents were able to see how much time the health care team spent in planning the care of their child. The PICU nurses commented that children had improved mood and fewer emotional outbursts when parents left the unit. Health care professionals were reminded that each child should be treated within the context of family and that parents bring valuable information to the treatment plan
Kuo et al, 2011	Despite widespread endorsement, PFCC continues to be insufficiently implemented into clinical practice	NA	Family-centered rounds are described as interdisciplinary rounds at the bedside in which patient and family share in the control of the management plan. Families specify that rounds are better when a nurse is present, when the family is introduced and involved in the discussion, and when medical terminology is avoided or interpreted	The advance of inpatient care shows that transformation to a fully family-centered system of care can begin with small changes. However, system-level changes must occur to enable providers and families to engage in information sharing and decision making, creating the partnership that leads to improved outcomes

Meert et al,[1] 2013	Endorsement and identification of benefits and risks of PFCC policies in PICU	NA	Patient-centered communication is the ideal process through which PFCC is implemented in daily practice	When applied to pediatric critical care, the key components of patient-centered communication are: addressing the patient's and family's perspective; understanding patients and families within their psychosocial context; involving patients and families in care to the extent they desire; reaching a shared understanding of the problem and agreeing on a treatment plan; and making decisions that are based on the best clinical evidence, consistent with patient and family values
Muething et al, 2007	Effects of inclusion of parents in bedside rounds	Single acute care unit at Cincinnati Children's Hospital	Family involvement seems to improve communication, shares decision making, and offers new learning for residents and students	Family-centered rounds increase the potential for more significant improvement for patient safety and improved clinical outcomes
Rosswurm et al,[8] 1999	Describe model to assist in synthesizing empirical and contextual evidence and integrating evidence-based changes into practice	NA	Practitioners need skills and resources to appraise, synthesize, and diffuse the best evidence into practice	Collaboration between researchers and practitioners within and among disciplines enhances the diffusion of evidence-based practice innovations

Abbreviation: NA, not available.

evidence-based practice, beginning with the assessment of the need for a change in practice, and ending with the integration of an evidence-based protocol.[8] This theoretic model is based on 6 distinct steps that guide practitioners to develop evidence-based changes in practice (**Fig. 2**).

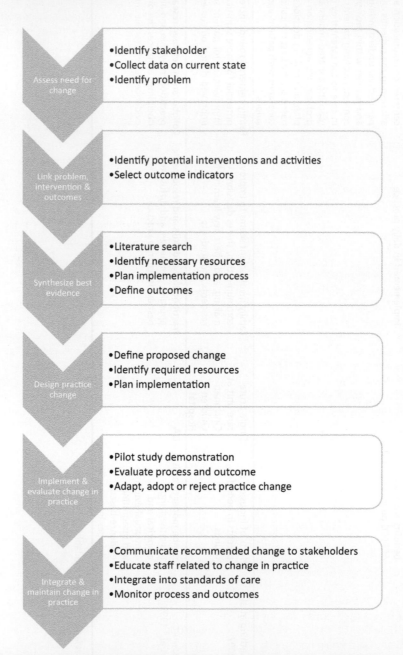

Fig. 2. Evidence-based practice model. (*Adapted from* Rosswurm MA, Larrabee JH. A model for change to evidence-based practice. Image J Nurs Sch 1999;31(4):318; with permission.)

METHODS
Setting

This project was conducted as a quality-improvement initiative in a 24-bed PICU of a pediatric tertiary care, academic medical center. During this project the PICU moved to a new tower and was expanded to a 36-bed PICU and a 12-bed cardiovascular ICU. The Clinical Scene Investigation (CSI) program provided by the American Association of Critical Care Nurses (AACN) began in June 2012 and continued with an Innovation Conference in September 2013. The implementation of this protocol began in January 2013 and the protocol remains in effect today.

ASSESSMENT AND PROBLEM IDENTIFICATION

A clinical nurse specialist (CNS) led this performance improvement project designed to improve patient/family understanding of the plan of care in the PICU. The CNS assessed the need for a change in practice; this assessment must include stakeholders and current data to support a need to change. The primary stakeholders in this process are the families, physicians, nursing staff, and other members of the health care team. The understanding that the family is at the heart of the solution is paramount. At the facility where this process was developed, families have been included in rounds for many years, but the awareness of their specific concerns and the follow-up to ensure they understood what was discussed had not previously been considered.

In the process of assessing and evaluating the needs of the patients, families, and other stakeholders, many project management tools were used, and the results shared with the staff to encourage their support and participation. Stakeholder diagrams (**Fig. 3**) and logic models (**Fig. 4**) were used to assess needs, develop short-term and long-term goals, and evaluate progress.

An exploration was conducted to assess the current practices related to interdisciplinary rounds in the PICU. During the exploration it was discovered that families were intermittently invited to rounds, without any explanation of the format or terminology used during rounds. Discussions were held with the parent advisory council to assess families' perceptions of interdisciplinary rounds and to understand what was helpful and what barriers existed. Results of discharge surveys sent to families were also evaluated to validate the findings from the discussions with the parent advisory council.

The assessment revealed that the families were not consistently invited to rounds and frequently did not understand what was discussed or the plan of care for their children. Discharge surveys were used to identify the current state of trust and confidence in nursing, the effectiveness of nursing communication, and the involvement with the family in the child's care; these metrics ranged from 74% to 78% (see **Fig. 1**). Several opportunities for improvement were identified from the assessment.

Interventions

Once the primary problems were identified, the team discussed them with the family advisory council and developed interventions to solve the underlying causes. Recognizing that the head-to-toe physiologic processes that rounding uses are not the normal thought process for families, the first intervention was directed at solving this problem. The first intervention begins within 24 hours of admission, with the bedside nurse explaining the process of rounds. This expectation was communicated to nursing with information related to PFCC and health literacy. The explanation for families included information related to the members of the interdisciplinary team,

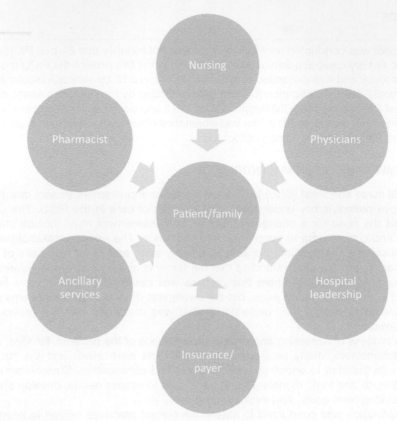

Fig. 3. Stakeholders.

the format of rounds, the discussions based on physiologic systems that permeate the rounding process, and the support provided to the family by the nursing staff.

A second intervention was developed to provide support for PFCC related to interdisciplinary rounds. This intervention includes daily prerounding and postrounding with the family by their child's nurse.

Outcome Measures/Data Collection

Outcome measures were chosen to evaluate the effectiveness of the protocol. These measures were based on results of discharge surveys obtained from National Research Corporation (NRC) and randomized questionnaires of parents currently in the PICU. The NRC collects, measures, analyzes, and reports multiple types of data across the continuum of care. One of the products provided by NRC are catalyst reports, also known as NRC Picker scores. These reports provide health care consumers' responses to specific questions for health care providers to evaluate changes in practice and care. Three questions from the discharge survey provided by NRC were closely related to this project. These questions were "How often did you have confidence and trust in the ICU nurses treating your child?"; "How often did the ICU nurses explain things in a way you could understand?"; and "How often did you have enough input or say in your child's care in the ICU?". Preimplementation data collected on these 3 questions showed a deficit, which we hypothesized would

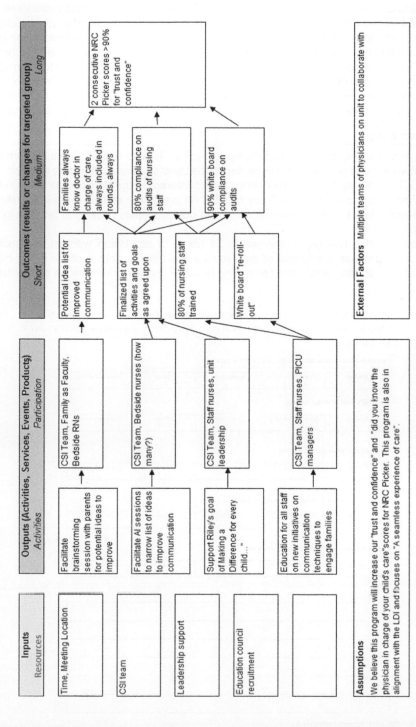

Program: **PICU: Partnerships in Care   Logic Model**
Situation: Making a Difference for every child, and every family it's what we do - and who I am"

Fig. 4. Logic model. AI, appreciative inquiry; LDI, leadership development institute; NRC, National Research Corporation; RN, registered nurse. (Copyright © by the Board of Regents of the University of Wisconsin System. All rights reserved.)

be alleviated by implementing this protocol. The 3 questions used for evaluation had preliminary rates ranging from 74% to 78%. These survey results validated what the parent advisory council told the team: they do not always understand what is said during rounds, they want to feel better informed, and they want to be involved in the care of their children. The randomized questionnaires were developed and analyzed by the CNS-led team to obtain quick answers to the most pressing questions (**Fig. 5**) in addition to the NRC Picker reports. This information became the catalyst for change, to improve the process of daily rounds and ensure that families understand the condition and plan for their children, and that their concerns are addressed on a daily basis.

Project Design

The new practice change was developed by the CNS-led team to increase families' involvement and comprehension related to the condition and plan of care for their children. The primary focus of the change was centered on the time period surrounding and including daily interdisciplinary rounds. As previously stated, there is significant evidence related to the communication and comprehension needs of families in the PICU.[4]

This practice change begins within 24 hours of admission with an explanation about the process and format of daily rounds and the importance of the family being a partner with the health care team. The practice change continues on a daily basis

In the Pediatric Intensive Care Unit, we want our families to be part of their child's care. You can help by telling us how well we explain your child's plan of care. Circle the answer next to each sentence that shows how you feel.

I know the doctor who is in charge of my child's care

Always	Most of the time	Sometimes	Never	Does not apply

My child's pain is under control

Always	Most of the time	Sometimes	Never	Does not apply

I am included in rounds every day

Always	Most of the time	Sometimes	Never	Does not apply

My questions are answered in a timely manner

Always	Most of the time	Sometimes	Never	Does not apply

I know the plan for my child's care every day

Always	Most of the time	Sometimes	Never	Does not apply

Comments:

Fig. 5. Parent questionnaire.

with the bedside nurse prerounding with the family to determine their questions and concerns. The bedside nurse discusses the patient's condition and the family's concerns with the family in the morning before rounds to determine whether there are any issues that the family would specifically like to discuss during rounds. The nurse then shares any concerns they planned to discuss during rounds with the family so that the family is not surprised by this information. The bedside nurse supports family members during rounds, ensuring that all of their questions are answered. The bedside nurse also works with the interdisciplinary team to evaluate the family's understanding of and comfort with the plan of care. During the time period following interdisciplinary rounds, the bedside nurse uses the teach-back method, in which the family is asked to explain to the bedside nurse what they heard during rounds using their own words.[9] This teach-back methodology provides the family with the opportunity to reflect on what they heard and to validate what they understood.[9] The final part of the teach-back methodology is completed once the family has relayed the information they heard during rounds. At this point the bedside nurse either confirms what was heard and understood or clarifies with further discussion with the family. The goal for the day is then written on a whiteboard in the patient's room to provide reassurance to the patient and family and to reinforce the goal for the day for the entire health care team.

Implementation and Evaluation

After the protocol was developed, an education plan for the PICU nursing staff was developed. Information related to PFCC, health literacy, and the shared goal of helping patients and families to be more effective partners in care was included. Education was provided in groups of 3 to 5 nurses with a PowerPoint presentation. Evidence-based resource materials were provided as part of this education, and were posted in the staff lounge for further study. The implementation date was celebrated with pizza parties for all the staff and gifts of badge holders and coffee cups with the "Partners in care united" logo were given to all staff. This event engaged the staff, emphasized the importance of the protocol, and increased staff awareness and expectations.

Specific metrics were used to evaluate progress toward the goal of improved communication between patients, families, and the health care team. These metrics were chosen based on their reliability and availability. It was determined that using the results of questionnaires sent to families after discharge from the hospital would provide the most global and reliable information.

Written questionnaires were also given to some families (see **Fig. 5**) while they were in the PICU. These questionnaires were used to assess how the protocol affected parents' perceptions and satisfaction while their children were still in the PICU.

RESULTS

The implementation of this protocol has resulted in improved patient satisfaction scores as shown by catalyst reports from NRC Picker (see **Fig. 1**). Evidence has also shown that improved communication and parental involvement is related to length of stay. During the 6 months following implementation of this process, length of stay reduced by 1 day. This change cannot be entirely attributed to this process, but it must be considered that this process had an impact on the reduced length of stay (**Fig. 6**). Anecdotally, PICU nurses reported increased satisfaction in being prepared to support families before, during, and after rounds. However, no metrics are available to provide quantitative data to support these reports.

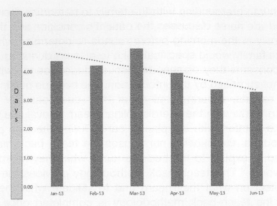

Fig. 6. Length of stay.

The comparison of preimplementation (74%–78%) and postimplementation data (86%–98%) shows improvements in each of the 3 test questions, ranging from 16% to 26%. The greatest improvement was seen in the question, "How often did the ICU nurses explain things in a way you could understand?" with a 26% increase from 78% to 98% (see **Fig. 1**).

A secondary metric that was used is a questionnaire (see **Fig. 5**) developed in house and distributed to 10 to 20 parents each month while they are in the PICU. This metric became the primary metric in late 2014, when the questions on the NRC Picker discharge survey were changed. The questionnaire initially provided an additional opportunity to gather data related to the effectiveness of the protocol, and this is now the primary metric to evaluate the protocol. Three of the items on this questionnaire are, "I am included in rounds every day"; "My questions are answered in a timely manner"; and "I know the plan for my child's care every day". The results of these questionnaires have shown an improvement from a starting low of 67% immediately after implementation and have sustained a rate of 87% or greater since the fifth month after implementation (**Fig. 7**).

The metrics used for evaluation were documented and analyzed each month to determine compliance toward the goal and evaluate the necessity for changes to

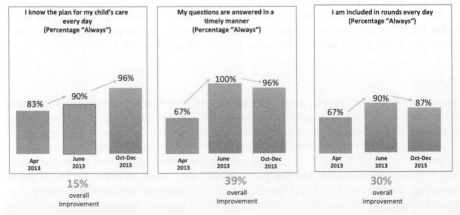

Fig. 7. Family questionnaire results.

the protocol. This information was initially shared with staff during huddles at the beginning of each shift and via postings in the report room and the staff lounge. Over time, the results were added to other reported unit metrics.

In accountable health care, patient satisfaction, outcomes, and financial benefits are of primary importance to health care systems. Although the effects of this protocol are difficult to identify in isolation from other activities occurring in the PICU, it is possible to estimate some realistic and potentially underestimated savings. When the pediatric Hospital Consumer Assessment of Healthcare Providers and Systems (HCAHPS) survey is implemented, it will be possible to determine the impact of patient satisfaction on reimbursement for Medicare patients.[10] Data from the hospital where this protocol was implemented show that the financial impact of improved patient satisfaction equates to $1358 per Medicare patient based on current Medicare reimbursement rates. Decreases in length of stay also have a significant financial impact. At the time this protocol was implemented in 2013, the cost to the hospital for a day in the PICU (room and board only) was $1542. The annual number of patients in the PICU was 2374, with an average length of stay of 3.8 days. This protocol has affected length of stay by a reduction of approximately 1 day, leading to potential annual cost savings of up to $3,660,708.

DISCUSSION

Results of this protocol were communicated to the PICU staff, the hospital Clinical Practice Council, the hospital system Professional Practice Steering Committee, the hospital system Evidence-Based Practice Council, and the hospital system chief nursing officer retreat. These presentations allowed a sharing of information with the intention of implementation of this protocol hospital-wide and eventually system-wide. This practice change has become the expected standard of care in the PICU. Sustainability for the project has been achieved through monthly feedback sessions related to successes, various contests related to knowledge of the protocol, and support from PICU and hospital leadership. The staff are proud of the work they are performing; the knowledge that this work is important to the patients and their families is a positive influence on sustainability. The data that have been analyzed provide positive evidence for the effectiveness of the practice changes developed through this quality-improvement project. Work based on this project continues to build sustainability and nurse satisfaction. Changes in the hospital system led to challenges in maintaining this process. By 2016, almost half of the PICU staff had less than 24 months' experience, which led to a need to develop a new training plan, to consistently prepare the new hires to effectively preround and postround with the families. Despite these challenges, the unit was able to maintain and sustain effectiveness over a 2.5-year period (see **Fig. 7**).

The use of the evidence-based practice theory provided a useful framework to assess the current state and necessity of the protocol, develop interventions based on current research and evidence, implement interventions, evaluate outcomes, and assess sustainability of changes in practice. This process supports the consistent use and diffusion of evidence-based practice.

Financial Investment

The financial costs for this project were larger than the anticipated costs required to replicate the results. This difference was caused by grant funding provided through the AACN as a CSI project. The $10,000 CSI grant was developed by AACN to empower staff nurses in creating unit-based change that is easily scaled hospital-wide. The CSI program was developed in response to IOM's report, *The Future of Nursing: Leading Change, Advancing Health*, which confirms the vital role nursing can play in the transformation of health care.[11]

The full financial costs for this project, including salaries, training, and promotional activities, were $9993 (**Table 2**). Specifically, this amount included the salaries of a CNS and 2 bedside nurses from the PICU to attend eight 6-hour change management classes provided by AACN. The cost also included the kick-off pizza parties, gifts for the staff, celebratory concession machine rentals, and prizes for sustainability contests. The cost of promotional materials, CSI training, and other expenses would not be necessary or potentially available to implement in an institution. Based on the budget provided by the grant from AACN and the funds that were consumed, it is estimated that costs to an institution will be less than $5000.

The literature matrix (see **Table 1**) provides necessary evidence and information in support of this protocol in other institutions. The time investment required would be best used in assessing current state, identifying metrics to evaluate outcomes, assessing feasibility, and the development of an education plan for staff.

IMPLICATIONS FOR THE CLINICAL NURSE SPECIALIST ROLE

This project incorporates the 3 spheres of influence designated by the National Association of Clinical Nurse Specialist (NACNS) as described in the organizational framework for CNS core competencies. These 3 spheres of influence include nurses/nursing practice, patients, and the health care organization or system.[12]

The CNS uses their collaboration skills in fulfilling the assessment of the quality and effectiveness of interdisciplinary communication and collaboration in relation to patients and their families during interdisciplinary rounds. This evidence-based protocol was developed in response to the assessment to achieve defined patient and system outcomes. This protocol also assists staff in the development of innovative, cost-effective programs or protocols of care while determining when the protocol or plan of care needs to be tailored to the individual.

Table 2 Financial cost of protocol			
Category	**Description**	**Expenses ($)**	**Remaining Balance ($)**
Total Budget			10,000
Salary and wages	Maximum allowed AACN classes and meeting time; could be more dependent on salary	5000	5000
Supplies			
Pizza party	Kick-off celebrations	640	4360
Badge holders and cups	Gifts for staff	1518	2842
Gift certificates	Prizes for competition to name parts of project	20	2822
Slushy machine	Celebration	315	2507
Work-out bags and pen lights	Gifts for staff	2500	7

Leadership for establishing, improving, and sustaining collaborative relationships to meet clinical needs is intricately woven into the metrics and feedback of this protocol. The CNS provided coaching and mentoring to advance the care of patients, families, groups of patients, and the profession of nursing, and this not only supported the protocol but also affected its success. Through the protocol the CNS and bedside registered nurse (RN) team led advanced skills training to address the problem of incomplete communication during interdisciplinary rounds in the PICU. Through multiple presentations, the evidence supporting this practice change and dissemination of outcomes has contributed to the advancement of the profession as a whole.

The CNS supported the analysis of research findings, application of evidence-based practice and quality improvement, and the effective implementation of research findings in clinical practice.

The role of the CNS is integral throughout the process of introducing patients/families to interdisciplinary rounding practice, prerounding with families to ensure that all concerns are brought forward during rounds, and postrounding with the families to ensure that they comprehend what was discussed during rounds. This protocol facilitates patient/family understanding of risks, benefits, and outcomes of the proposed health care regimen to promote informed decision making. It also promotes the facilitation of resolution of ethical conflicts, and fosters professional accountability in self and others. The continued use of this protocol supports the patients/families, the bedside nurses, and the entire interdisciplinary team in better communication, which translates into improved patient satisfaction and outcomes.[4]

SUMMARY

PFCC is a recognized and supported standard in health care. In pediatrics, the support of parents during daily rounds has been attempted many times and in multiple ways. The necessity to further improve communication and comprehension for parents with a child in the PICU is an accepted fact. This protocol was developed to not only improve the parents' inclusion and comprehension during rounds but to also better prepare them by explaining the rounding process and terminology, prerounding to ensure that all of the families' questions are answered during daily rounds, postrounding to assess what the families heard in rounds and provide appropriate clarification, and posting the goal for the day in the room for the health care team and parents/patients to see.

The implementation of this evidence-based protocol has had a significant impact on patients, families, and hospital staff in the PICU at Riley Hospital for Children. Benefits to patients, families, and hospital staff are shown in the way patient/family satisfaction has improved, patient length of stay has decreased, and satisfaction of hospital staff has increased as they realize the potential they have to improve the patients and families' care. What started out as an idea to improve families' involvement and understanding related to their children's care has provided many additional positive results and has become a standard of practice in the PICU at Riley Hospital for Children.

ACKNOWLEDGMENTS

The authors acknowledge the AACN for their investment in the CSI project that funded this project. Connie Neuzerling RN, Susan Willock RN, and Jen Blevins RN for their dedication to help develop and implement this process. Tracie Hart RN and Patricia Stanifer RN for their dedication in helping to sustain this project. The leadership at Riley Hospital for Children, and specifically the PICU at Riley Hospital for Children, for the support to bring ideas from the bedside to life.

REFERENCES

1. Meert KL, Clark J, Eggley S. Family-centered care in the pediatric intensive care unit. Pediatr Clin North Am 2013;60(3):761–72.
2. Committee on Quality of Health Care in America. Crossing the quality chasm: a new health system for the 21st century. Washington, DC: Institute of Medicine; 2001. Crossing the Quality Chasm.
3. Committee on Hospital Care and Institute for Patient-and Family-Centered Care. Policy statement: patient-and family-centered care and the pediatrician's role. Pediatrics 2012;129(2):394–404.
4. Kleiber C, Davenport T, Freyenberger B. Open bedside rounds for families with children in pediatric intensive care units. Am J Crit Care 2006;15(5):492–6.
5. Jacobowski NL, Girard TD, Mulder JA, et al. Communication in critical care: family rounds in the intensive care unit. Am J Crit Care 2010;19(5):421–30.
6. Davidson JE. Family-centered care meeting the needs of patients' families and helping families adapt to critical illness. Crit Care Nurse 2009;29(3):28–34.
7. Shelton W, Moore CD, Socaris S, et al. The effect of a family support intervention on family satisfaction, length-of-stay, and cost of care in the intensive care unit. Crit Care Med 2010;38(5):1315–20.
8. Rosswurm MA, Larrabee JH. A model for change to evidence-based practice. Image J Nurs Sch 1999;31(4):317–22.
9. Tamura-Lis W. Teach-back for quality education and patient safety. Urol Nurs 2013;33(6):267–71, 298.
10. Centers for Medicare & Medicaid Services. HCAHPS: patients' perspectives of care survey. CMS.gov; 2014. Available at: https://www.cms.gov/Medicare/Quality-Initiatives-Patient-Assessment-instruments/HospitalQualityInits/HospitalHCAHPS.html. Accessed July 18, 2016.
11. Committee on the Robert Wood Johnson Foundation Initiative on the Future of Nursing, at the Institute of Medicine. The future of nursing: leading change, advancing health. Washington, DC: The National Academies Press; 2011.
12. National Association of Clinical Nurse Specialists. Clinical nurse specialist core competencies executive summary. Philadelphia: National CNS Competency Task Force; 2010. CNS Core Competencies.

Continuous Capnography in Pediatric Intensive Care

Christine M. Riley, BS, MSN, APRN, CPNP-AC

KEYWORDS

- Capnography • Pediatric • Critical care • End-tidal CO_2

KEY POINTS

- Continuous capnography monitoring has a variety of uses in the pediatric intensive care setting.
- Capnography allows for noninvasive continuous monitoring of airway, breathing, and circulation in critically ill pediatric patients.
- Monitoring of physiologic dead space via arterial carbon dioxide and end-tidal carbon dioxide gradient has important diagnostic and prognostic implications in pediatric intensive care patients.
- Capnography has diagnosis-specific applications for pediatric patients with congenital heart disease, reactive airway disease, neurologic emergencies, and metabolic derangement.

INTRODUCTION

Capnography or end-tidal carbon dioxide ($Etco_2$) monitoring has a variety of uses in the pediatric intensive care setting. The ability to continuously measure exhaled carbon dioxide can provide critical information about cardiac and pulmonary function in addition to confirming accuracy of invasive airway placement. This monitoring modality has become standard of care in many intensive care areas.[1] This article reviews the basic principles and clinical applications of $Etco_2$ monitoring in the pediatric intensive care unit (PICU).

Principals of Continuous End-tidal Monitoring

Basic physiology

Capnometry refers to the measurement of carbon dioxide (CO_2) exhaled by a patient and capnography is a visual representation of exhaled CO_2 graphically as a function of tidal volume or time.[2] Noninvasive measurement of CO_2 has many practical

Disclosure: The author has nothing to disclose.
Division of Cardiac Critical Care Medicine, Children's National Health System, 111 Michigan Avenue, Washington, DC 20010, USA
E-mail address: criley@childrensnational.org

Table 1	
Continuous capnography in pediatric critical care	
Uses of Continuous Capnography in Pediatric Critical Care	
Airway	• ETT placement confirmation during intubation • Monitor for artificial airway displacement or obstruction • Improve safety during interhospital transport • Monitor patency of natural airway during conscious sedation
Breathing	• Evaluation adequacy of ventilation • Noninvasive titration of ventilatory support • Evaluation of physiologic dead space and V/Q matching • Monitor alterations in airway resistance in reactive airway disease
Circulation	• Monitor changes in cardiac output • Monitor degree of pulmonary blood flow in cyanotic heart disease • Goal directed evaluation of CPR quality during resuscitation • Monitor for ROSC during resuscitation
Additional	• Evaluate for changes in metabolic rate • Monitor decreased cerebral blood flow in TBI • Enteral feeding tube placement

Abbreviations: CPR, cardiopulmonary resuscitation; ETT, endotracheal tube; ROSC, return of spontaneous circulation; TBI, traumatic brain injury.

applications in the PICU, including real-time assessment of airway, breathing, and circulation (**Table 1**).

The tissues produce carbon dioxide as a byproduct of aerobic metabolism. Clinical conditions that increase tissue metabolic rate (ie, fever, trauma, sepsis) increase production of carbon dioxide. Conditions that decrease tissue metabolic rates (ie, sedation, hypothermia, and paralysis) decrease the production of carbon dioxide.

CO_2 diffuses through the tissues into the blood stream, where it binds to hemoglobin and is carried to the lungs, to be exchanged for oxygen and exhaled. Only areas of the lung that are perfused by the blood stream participate in gas exchange (alveolar ventilation). Areas of the lung that are not able to exchange gas with the blood stream are considered dead-space. Minute ventilation, the amount of gas moved through the airways each minute, is the sum of alveolar and dead-space ventilation times the respiratory rate. Anatomic dead space occurs in all patients, because there are parts of the airway solely dedicated to the movement of air toward the terminal bronchioles and alveoli. Physiologic dead space can occur in addition to anatomic dead space because the ratio of blood flow to ventilation varies between lung units. Ventilation/perfusion ratio or V/Q matching describes the adequacy of matching ventilated areas of the lung with perfused areas of the lung. Areas of the lung that are ventilated but not well perfused are considered physiologic dead space. Areas that are perfused but not ventilated are considered interpulmonary shunts. All areas of the lung are between these two extremes. Disease conditions can further alter the degree of V/Q matching by increasing physiologic dead space.[3] Comparison of the amount of CO_2 exhaled with the amount of CO_2 in arterial blood allows an estimation of V/Q matching. This gradient, known as $Paco_2$-$Petco_2$, is about 4 to 7 mm Hg under normal conditions, but increases in conditions that adversely affect V/Q matching and decreases as V/Q matching improves.[2]

The concentration of CO_2 in exhaled gas varies depending on the metabolic rate of the tissues, amount of alveolar ventilation, and amount of pulmonary blood flow.

Critically ill pediatric patients often have disorders that result in alterations of V/Q matching (eg, lung disease or low cardiac output), so monitoring $Paco_2$-$Petco_2$ is useful in addition to capnography when integrated with other pertinent patient data.

Types of measurement

CO_2 concentration in a sample of exhaled gas is measured via infrared absorption.[4] There are 2 main types of devices: mainstream or in-line, in which a sensor is connected to an endotracheal tube directly as part of the breathing circuit; or sidestream, which continuously draws a sample of exhaled gas via a nasal cannula.[5] Mainstream measurement devices provide rapid analysis without pulling from tidal volumes, but the devices are typically bulkier. Sidestream devices are typically less bulky and can be used in nonintubated patients, but create a small leak from the breathing circuit and a small delay in sample analysis.[6] A normal capnogram (**Fig. 1**) starts as gas exits the dead space, giving a baseline measurement of zero, then the value rapidly increases as gas is released from the intermediate airways. A plateau is seen on the curve as gas moves from the alveoli, followed by a rapid decline as the next breath is inhaled. Changes in the gas waveform as well as the actual value are useful in clinical management decisions (**Table 2**).

DISCUSSION

There are many clinical applications for continuous capnography in pediatric critical care.[7] These applications can be grouped into the following framework: airway, breathing, circulation, and diagnosis specific.

Clinical Applications

Airway
Capnography at the time of intubation ensures endotracheal rather than esophageal tube placement. Capnography is more reliable in this situation than other methods of airway placement confirmation, including auscultation, and is independent of provider experience level.[8,9] It can also be used to monitor for tube displacement or obstruction in ventilated patients, providing an additional safety monitor in the critical care setting. Intrahospital transport of intubated critical care patients to diagnostic and procedural areas can create potential for instability or artificial airway displacement, making $Etco_2$ monitoring an important safety feature in these situations.[10,11] The American Society of Anesthesiologists has considered capnography

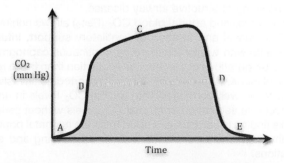

Fig. 1. Normal capnogram. A: Gas exits the dead space giving a baseline measurement of zero. B: Rapid increase as gas is released from the intermediate airways. C: Plateau is seen on the curve as gas moves from the alveoli. D: Rapid decline as the next breath is inhaled. E: Return to baseline.

Table 2
Capnography waveforms and clinical correlations

Wave Form	Clinical Correlation
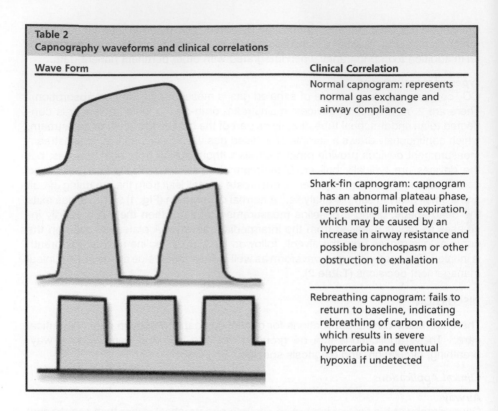	Normal capnogram: represents normal gas exchange and airway compliance
	Shark-fin capnogram: capnogram has an abnormal plateau phase, representing limited expiration, which may be caused by an increase in airway resistance and possible bronchospasm or other obstruction to exhalation
	Rebreathing capnogram: fails to return to baseline, indicating rebreathing of carbon dioxide, which results in severe hypercarbia and eventual hypoxia if undetected

a standard of care for anesthetic monitoring since 1986 and recommends tube confirmation by capnography in the 2013 practice guidelines for management of difficult airways.[12] Capnography can also be used to monitor protection of the natural airway and avoidance of hypopnea during conscious sedation using a sidestream device connected to a nasal cannula.

Breathing

Capnography values, trends, and waveforms can be used in the pediatric critical care setting to assess the adequacy of ventilation, detect physiologic dead space, and as an indicator of worsening obstructive airway disease.

The correlation of $Etco_2$ and arterial blood CO_2 (Pao_2) allows noninvasive real-time monitoring of CO_2 removal and titration of ventilatory support. Intubated pediatric intensive care patients who were monitored by continuous capnography have been shown to have shorter durations of mechanical ventilation than those receiving routine clinical management alone.[13] Tai and colleagues[14] reported noninvasive capnography via nasal cannula to be well correlated with arterial CO_2 levels in unintubated neonates, allowing accurate estimation of arterial CO_2 levels without serial arterial blood gas sampling. This finding is particularly important in the neonatal population because arterial blood sampling in this population can be challenging and associated with serious complications.

Estimation of physiologic dead space can be monitored by $Paco_2$-$Petco_2$ gradient and is important in pediatric critical care patients for prognostic and therapeutic reasons. Physiologic dead space occurs when areas of the lung are ventilated but do not participate in gas exchange because they lack adequate perfusion. Physiologic dead space often increases in critical illness as part of primary disorders like lung disease or secondary to other disorders, such as low cardiac output or alveolar overdistension. Patients with large amounts of physiologic dead space are at risk for failed extubation, longer duration of ventilator support, and increased mortality.[14–17] Titrating ventilator support to minimize dead space has been shown to improve outcomes in children with respiratory failure.[18–20] Bhalla and colleagues[21] showed that estimation of physiologic dead space using capnography was highly correlated with other more detailed methods of physiologic dead-space management in intubated children without hypoxemia, allowing easily attainable bedside estimation of improving or worsening condition. Infants undergoing stage 1 palliation for single-ventricle congenital heart disease were noted to have an increase in pulmonary dead space following the procedure and those with higher dead-space fraction (calculated by $Paco_2$-$Petco_2$ gradient) in the first 48 hours postoperatively had longer durations of mechanical ventilation and hospital length of stay.[22]

Changes in capnography tracings or values may indicate changes in airway resistance, alveolar compliance, or inadequate ventilatory support. The capnography waveform in obstructive airway disease is typically a sloped graph or shark-fin shape rather than square.[5] If ventilator settings are preventing complete exhalation or "air trapping" the capnography graph does not return to baseline, indicating rebreathing and inadequate CO_2 removal.[5] Changes in capnography waveform and their clinical correlations are shown in **Table 2**. A study of delayed sternal closures in pediatric patients following cardiac surgery reported a decrease in both tidal volume and $Etco_2$ by 17% and 29% respectively.[23] These changes reflect decreases in alveolar ventilation secondary to a decrease in respiratory compliance and show the utility of $Etco_2$ monitoring for respiratory mechanics. Continuous $Etco_2$ allows titration of ventilator support by monitoring for adequate CO_2 removal without frequent arterial blood gas samples. Rowan and colleagues[24] reported a 40% reduction in arterial blood gas samples over a 6-month period following implementation of continuous capnography, providing significant cost-savings.

Circulation

$Etco_2$ is a useful measure of circulation and cardiac output as blood is consistently delivered to the lungs carrying carbon dioxide. Alterations in cardiac output decrease pulmonary blood flow therefore also decreasing exhaled carbon dioxide. This makes $Etco_2$ particularly useful during cardiopulmonary resuscitation (CPR) and when caring for children with congenital heart disease.

Cardiopulmonary resuscitation The American Heart Association 2015 guidelines for the resuscitation of children include the use of continuous capnography for intubated patients receiving CPR.[25] Continuous capnography in this patient population allows providers to monitor the quality of CPR, optimize chest compressions, and assess for return of spontaneous circulation in addition to confirmation of endotracheal tube placement. Studies of the use of capnography in cardiac arrest have shown that $Etco_2$ of greater than 15 mm Hg is associated with return of spontaneous circulation (ROSC),[1,25] allowing continuous capnography to be used for target-directed therapy and as a prognostic indicator.

Pulmonary blood flow and estimation of cardiac output Exhaled CO_2 mirrors the amount of pulmonary blood flow, making this monitoring modality particularly useful in intensive care units caring for children with congenital heart disease. Numerous studies have shown that the $Paco_2$-$Petco_2$ gradient is increased in children with cyanotic heart disease but minimal in acyanotic patients.[26–28] Even though the numeric $Etco_2$ values are not as closely associated, the trend and the $Paco_2$-$PEtco_2$ gradient are very valuable. Should there be an alteration in pulmonary blood flow, either secondary to anatomic changes such as shunt occlusion or ductal narrowing or secondary to decreases in cardiac output, a widening $Paco_2$-$PEtco_2$ gradient may be observed before there is a change in hemodynamics or saturation.[29] Low $Etco_2$ values or changes in $Paco_2$-$PEtco_2$ gradient in patient with shunted cyanotic heart disease warrants rapid investigation for this reason.

Capnography is a useful adjunct to heart rate and blood pressuring monitoring as $Etco_2$ mirrors cardiac output. Capnography in healthy children has been shown to be comparable with Fick method calculations.[30] The correlation of capnography values and $Paco_2$-$PEtco_2$ gradient with important change in pulmonary blood flow and cardiac output is particularly important to understand and monitor in the pediatric ICU, especially in patients with congenital heart disease, for whom the ICU setting functions as an extension of the operating room.

Diagnosis specific

In addition to monitoring for abnormalities in airway, breathing, and circulation in pediatric intensive care patients, continuous capnography provides additional monitoring for certain diagnoses commonly encountered in the pediatric ICU.

Patients with respiratory distress benefit from capnography because abnormal waveforms and values provide noninvasive information on the adequacy of ventilation and airway compliance. Children with moderate to severe respiratory distress secondary to asthma, bronchiolitis, and pneumonia were found to have high levels of correlation between $Etco_2$ and venous CO_2, supporting noninvasive monitoring in these conditions.[31] In addition, changes in airway compliance and degree of obstruction are reflected in continuous capnogram, allowing additional monitoring in patients prone to bronchospasm, as in reactive airway disease.[4]

Children with traumatic brain injury are particularly sensitive to changes in $Paco_2$ because this value also dramatically affects cerebral blood flow. Hypocapnia-induced cerebral vasoconstriction alters blood flow to the brain and creates regional decreases in oxygen delivery, which may exacerbate neurologic conditions by causing secondary ischemia.[32] Bagwell and colleagues[33] showed that children with neurologic emergencies who had $Etco_2$ values of less than 30 mm Hg had a significant decrease in cerebral blood flow and regional tissue oxygenation. They concluded that capnography is particularly useful in the resuscitation of this patient population because it allows monitoring of inadvertent and potentially detrimental hyperventilation.

Children admitted with diabetic ketoacidosis (DKA) benefit from capnography as a noninvasive monitor of metabolic status. Carbon dioxide is a byproduct of aerobic metabolism so alterations in the level of CO_2 indicate alterations in metabolic rate. Pediatric patients with DKA often present with compensatory hyperventilation, which improves as their metabolic derangement normalizes and serum pH returns to baseline. Garcia and colleagues[34] found that $PEtco_2$ provided an accurate estimate of $Paco_2$ values in children with DKA, allowing continuous monitoring of metabolic state by capnography in this patient population.

SUMMARY

Continuous capnography has a variety of uses in the pediatric critical care population in addition to confirmation of endotracheal tube placement and has become considered the standard of care in this setting. When integrated with other pertinent patient data, including physical assessment, capnography can provide valuable real-time information on patient status, including amount of physiologic dead space, adequacy of ventilatory support, sufficiency of V/Q matching, and variations in pulmonary blood flow/cardiac output.

REFERENCES

1. Sivarajan VB, Bohn D. Monitoring of standard hemodynamic parameters: heart rate, systemic blood pressure, atrial pressure, pulse oximetry, and end-tidal CO_2. Pediatr Crit Care Med 2011;12(4 Suppl):S2–11.
2. Sullivan KJ, Kissoon N, Goodwin SR. End-tidal carbon dioxide monitoring in pediatric emergencies. Pediatr Emerg Care 2005;21(5):327–32.
3. Cheifetz IM, Venkataraman ST, Hamel DS. Respiratory monitoring. In: Nichols DG, editor. Rogers' textbook of pediatric intensive care. 4th edition. Baltimore (MD): Lippincott Williams & Wilkins; 2008. p. 662–87.
4. Briening E. End-tidal carbon dioxide measurement. In: Verger J, Lebet R, editors. AACNs procedure manual for pediatric acute and critical care. Philadelphia: Elsevier; 2008. p. 121–40.
5. Cortez E, Ganesan R. Pulmonary disorders. In: Reuter-Rice K, Bolick B, editors. Pediatric acute care: a guide for interprofessional practice. Burlington (VT): Jones and Bartlett; 2012. p. 995–1090.
6. Cheifetz IM, Myers TR. Respiratory therapies in the critical care setting. Should every mechanically ventilated patient be monitored with capnography from intubation to extubation? Respir Care 2007;52(4):423–38 [discussion: 438–42].
7. Eipe N, Doherty DR. A review of pediatric capnography. J Clin Monit Comput 2010;24(4):261–8.
8. Birmingham PK, Cheney FW, Ward RJ. Esophageal intubation: a review of detection techniques. Anesth Analg 1986;65(8):886–91.
9. Knapp S, Kofler J, Stoiser B, et al. The assessment of four different methods to verify tracheal tube placement in the critical care setting. Anesth Analg 1999;88(4):766–70.
10. Tobias JD, Lynch A, Garrett J. Alterations of end-tidal carbon dioxide during the intrahospital transport of children. Pediatr Emerg Care 1996;12(4):249–51.
11. Bhende MS, Karr VA, Wiltsie DC, et al. Evaluation of a portable infrared end-tidal carbon dioxide monitor during pediatric interhospital transport. Pediatrics 1995; 95(6):875–8.
12. American Society of Anesthesiologists Task Force on Management of the Difficult Airway. Practice guidelines for management of the difficult airway: update by the American Society of Anesthesiologists Task Force on Management of the Difficult Airway. Anesthesiology 2003;98(5):1269–77.
13. Hamel D, Cheifetz I. Continuous monitoring of volumetric capnography reduces length of mechanical ventilation in a heterogeneous group of pediatric ICU patients. Respir Care 2005;50(11):1517.
14. Tai CC, Lu FL, Chen PC, et al. Noninvasive capnometry for end-tidal carbon dioxide monitoring via nasal cannula in nonintubated neonates. Pediatr Neonatol 2010;51(6):330–5.
15. Hubble CL, Gentile MA, Tripp DS, et al. Deadspace to tidal volume ration predicts successful extubation in infants and children. Crit Care Med 2000;28(6):2034–40.
16. Ong T, Stuart-Killion RB, Daniel BM, et al. Higher pulmonary dead space may predict prolonged mechanical ventilation after cardiac surgery. Pediatr Pulmonol 2009;44(5):457–63.
17. Nuckton TJ, Alonso JA, Kallet RH, et al. Pulmonary dead-space fraction as a risk factor for death in the acute respiratory distress syndrome. N Engl J Med 2002; 346(17):1281–6.

18. Ghuman AK, Newth CJ, Khemani RG. The association between the end tidal alveolar dead space fraction and mortality in pediatric acute hypoxemic respiratory failure. Pediatr Crit Care Med 2012;13(1):11–5.

19. Fengmei G, Jin C, Songqiao L, et al. Dead space fraction changes during PEEP titration following lung recruitment in patients with ARDS. Respir Care 2010; 57(10):1578–85.

20. Yang Y, Huang Y, Tang R, et al. Optimization of positive end-expiratory pressure by volumetric capnography variables in lavage-induced acute lung injury. Respiration 2014;87(1):75–83.

21. Bhalla AK, Rubin S, Newth CJ, et al. Monitoring dead space in mechanically ventilated children: volumetric capnography verse time-based capnography. Respir Care 2015;60(11):1548–55.

22. Shakti D, McElhinney DB, Gauvreau K, et al. Pulmonary deadspace and postoperative outcomes in neonates undergoing stage 1 palliation operation for single ventricle heart disease. Pediatr Crit Care Med 2014;15(8):728–34.

23. Main E, Elliott MJ, Schindler M, et al. Effect of delayed sternal closure after cardiac surgery on respiratory function in ventilated infants. Crit Care Med 2001; 29:1798–802.

24. Rowan CM, Speicher RH, Hedlund T, et al. Implementation of continuous capnography is associated with a decreased utilization of blood gases. J Clin Med Res 2015;7(2):71–5.

25. Atkins DL, Berger S, Duff JP, et al. Part 11: pediatric basic life support and cardiopulmonary resuscitation quality: 2015 American Heart Association guidelines update for cardiopulmonary resuscitation and emergency cardiovascular care (reprint). Pediatrics 2015;136(Suppl 2):S167–75.

26. Wilson J, Russo P, Russo J, et al. Noninvasive monitoring of carbon dioxide in infants and children with congenital heart disease: end-tidal verse transcutaneous techniques. J Intensive Care Med 2005;20:291–5.

27. Fletcher R. The relationship between the arterial to end-tidal PCO_2 difference and hemoglobin saturation in patients with congenital heart disease. Anesthesiology 1991;75:210–6.

28. Short JA, Paris ST, Booker PD, et al. Arterial to end-tidal carbon dioxide tension difference in children with congenital heart disease. Br J Anaesth 2001;86:349–53.

29. Schuller JL, Bovill JG, Nijveld A. End-tidal carbon dioxide concentration as an indicator of pulmonary blood flow during closed heart surgery in children. A report of two cases. Br J Anaesth 1985;57:1257–9.

30. Pianosi P, Hochman J. End-tidal estimates of arterial PCO_2 for cardiac output measurement by CO_2 rebreathing: a study in patients with cystic fibrosis and healthy controls. Pediatr Pulmonol 1996;22:154–60.

31. Moses JM, Alexander JL, Agus MS. The correlation and level of agreement between end-tidal and blood gas pCO_2 in children with respiratory distress: a retrospective analysis. BMC Pediatr 2009;9:20.

32. Meng L, Gelb AW. Regulation of cerebral autoregulation by carbon dioxide. Anesthesiology 2015;122(1):196–205.

33. Bagwell TA, Abramo TJ, Albert GW, et al. Cerebral oximetry with blood volume index and capnography in intubated and hyperventilated patients. Am J Emerg Med 2016;34(6):1102–7.

34. Garcia E, Abramo TJ, Okada P, et al. Capnometry for noninvasive continuous monitoring of metabolic status in pediatric diabetic ketoacidosis. Crit Care Med 2003;31(10):2539–43.

Massive Transfusion Protocol Simulation
An Innovative Approach to Team Training

Allison Langston, BSN, RN[a], Dayna Downing, MHA, MBA[b],*,
Jennifer Packard, MBA, MT (ASCP), SBB[c], Marion Kopulos, MSN, RN-BC[d,e],
Shelley Burcie, BSN, RN[f], Kay Martin, BSRC, RRT-NPS[g],
Brennan Lewis, MSN, RN, CPNP-PC/AC, PCNS-BC[h]

KEYWORDS

- Hemorrhage • Simulation training • Blood bank • Spinal fusion
- Crisis resource management • Massive Transfusion Protocol

KEY POINTS

- Massive transfusion for severe hemorrhage requires closed-loop communication.
- Proper closed-loop communication mitigates risk, increasing patient safety.
- Simulation education training helps prepare staff for high-risk low-probability events.
- Interdisciplinary simulation education training improves processes and closed-loop communication.

INTRODUCTION

A life-threatening hemorrhage requiring massive transfusion can occur in a variety of clinical situations, including unexpected intraoperative and postoperative hemorrhages, as well as traumatic injuries and extracorporeal membrane oxygenation.[1] It is associated

Disclosure Statement: The authors have no commercial or financial conflicts of interest and have not received any funding sources.
[a] Quality, Children's Health, Children's Medical Center, 1935 Medical District Drive, Dallas, TX 75235, USA; [b] Simulation Lab, Children's Health, Children's Medical Center, 1935 Medical District Drive, Dallas, TX 75235, USA; [c] Transfusion and Tissue Service, Children's Health, Children's Medical Center, 1935 Medical District Drive, Dallas, TX 75235, USA; [d] Emergency Department and Intensive Care Unit, Children's Health, Children's Medical Center, 7601 Preston Road, Plano, TX 75024, USA; [e] Emergency Department and Intensive Care Unit, Children's Health, Children's Medical Center, 1935 Medical District Drive, Dallas, TX 75235, USA; [f] Critical Care Services, Children's Health, Children's Medical Center, 1935 Medical District Drive, Dallas, TX 75235, USA; [g] Simulation Program, Children's Health, Children's Medical Center, 1935 Medical District Drive, Dallas, TX 75235, USA; [h] Patient Education and Engagement, Children's Health, Children's Medical Center, 1935 Medical District Drive, Dallas, TX 75235, USA
* Corresponding author.
E-mail address: Dayna.Downing@childrens.com

Crit Care Nurs Clin N Am 29 (2017) 259–269
http://dx.doi.org/10.1016/j.cnc.2017.01.011
0899-5885/17/© 2017 Elsevier Inc. All rights reserved.
ccnursing.theclinics.com

with significant mortality and morbidity, making a rapidly organized response to the massive hemorrhage critical to improve outcomes.[2] Massive Transfusion Protocols (MTPs) are used in many facilities to ensure a rapid and efficient response to patients with substantial uncontrolled blood loss. To maximize patient safety and improve outcomes, an organized systematic response to a patient with a critical massive hemorrhage requiring massive transfusion needs to be practiced with the team of health care professionals, to ensure clear communication and teamwork.

BACKGROUND

As services at a 72-bed pediatric facility began expanding, a need for organized training came to light. These services included performing spinal fusion surgeries to correct idiopathic scoliosis in the pediatric population. There is a high risk of postoperative hemorrhage, when performing corrective spinal fusion surgery and a need for initiation of MTP may arise. As the facility was planning for the new spinal fusion surgeries, a decision was made to plan a collaborative approach to education and preparation, by using simulation.

The Institute of Medicine's publication *To Err is Human: Building a Better Health System* recommended simulation as one of the interdisciplinary team training initiatives to assist in combating the astonishingly high number of medical errors in the United States.[3] Health care simulation depicts a clinical environment that allows the provider to be immersed in the re-creation of an event with the "intent to practice, educate, or test systems, and/or human actions and movement."[4] Simulations that mimic work environments and patient encounters create opportunities for hands-on learning in a safe, risk-free environment. This has become the desired method of learning, rendering the concept of "see one, do one, teach one" on patients outdated and impractical.[5]

Immediately after the simulation, participants engage in a "debriefing or after-action review," driven by the goals of reflection, analysis, and synthesis in an effort to eliminate points of failure at the participant and systems levels.[6] By replicating high-risk low-probability clinical events, such as MTP, staff can examine human factors and systems processes to increase patient safety. One of the greatest benefits of simulation is the ability to practice procedures, aiming for perfection while improving processes without putting patients at risk.[7]

Pediatric patients with spinal fusion who are hemorrhaging may need to be stabilized in the pediatric intensive care unit (PICU) using the level 1 rapid infuser and the MTP, with which many are not familiar.[8] At this facility, MTP is based on patient weight and aims to prevent dilutional coagulopathy by providing a set ratio of blood products to the patient (**Table 1**).[9]

The blood products are provided in packs. Each pack contains the same number of blood components and is designed to be completely transfused before transfusing products from subsequent packs. Because of the serious nature and the intensity of the patient requiring the MTP, simulation of the event was determined to be one of the most effective ways to prepare, measure readiness, and highlight areas for improvement.

Finally, by using simulation as an educational adjunct, participants are more likely to retain the information given during the didactic portion of the training. Looking at simulation through the lens of Bloom's Taxonomy, simulation puts participants in situations in which they must demonstrate not only that they can recall the material of the lecture, but that they can understand the information to the point of applying it properly to the situation in which they find themselves.[10] During the debriefing phase, they take their

Table 1 Ratio of products provided for MTP	
Patient Weight, kg	**Blood Components Provided in Each Pack**
<10	1:1 ratio of packed red blood cells (PRBCs), thawed plasma, and apheresis platelets
10–40	2 PRBCs, 1 thawed plasma, 1 apheresis platelet 5 Cryoprecipitate for 2nd and 4th packs
>40	5 PRBCs, 3 thawed plasma, 1 apheresis platelet 10 Cryoprecipitate for 2nd and 4th packs

From Children's Health System of Texas (2016). Massive Transfusion Protocol. Published internal document; with permission.

understanding a step further to being able to logically think through their actions and, in some cases, validate their actions, or recognize their knowledge gaps.

METHOD
Collaboration in Education Planning

The education preparation began by scheduling a planning committee meeting with the subject matter experts from the PICU, blood bank, and simulation program to discuss creating a scenario to help prepare staff for the activation of the MTP on an actual patient. The first obstacle is for staff to identify when to activate MTP. Research does not clearly define the amount of blood loss that warrants MTP to be initiated.[1] The massive transfusion process needs to be activated when a patient's blood loss occurs faster than the clinical bedside staff's ability to replace it using the traditional transfusion process. The simulation objectives were determined by the established learning needs of the participants. The MTP scenario was considered a low-probability high-risk scenario and was designed as an event that could occur with the patient population with new spinal fusion. Staff needed to demonstrate closed-loop communication and organization required to effectively carry out the MTP in a clinical setting.

Simulation Objectives

- Recognize the indications for and the principles related to MTP
- Demonstrate situational awareness and teamwork
- Demonstrate the principles of crisis resource management

Scenario Preparation

The location was determined by the planning committee to occur in the PICU with the intent to test the MTP process with staff in the actual environment that it would take place. This allows staff to work through their work flow process, resource man agement, and role recognition. The time of day of the scenario activation was determined by staff's availability for training. The participants were notified that a scenario of MTP was going to be performed after a scheduled didactic course preparing them to care for the postoperative spinal fusion surgery patient. During the scenario, adjuncts were introduced to make the scenario as relevant as possible, including the following:

- Utilization of equipment
  - Level 1 rapid infuser
  - Enflow infuser

- ○ Intravenous tubing and pump
- ○ Bair hugger
- ○ iSTAT (Abbott Point of Care, NJ), glucometer, and Hemocue (HemoCue America, CA): point-of-care testing (POCT)
- ○ Code medications
- • Proper use of personal protective equipment
- • Communication within the interdisciplinary team
- • Real-time event documentation

The laboratory and blood bank staff prepared for the massive transfusion simulation by training extensively on the MTP. An existing massive transfusion model from the larger acute care facility within the same health care system was applied to this location. Intradepartmental mock scenarios and direct observation of staff members were used to ensure staff was aware of how to perform the processes required when a massive transfusion event occurred. In the days before the facility simulation event, the blood bank prepared mock expired blood products to be dispensed. All mock blood products were made with unique labels so that the transfusion service could crossmatch and dispense the blood products using the computer system. Sufficient mock products were prepared to allow the simulation patient to receive 2 massive transfusion packs.

Communication and Organization

Activation of MTP must be performed via concise communication to the blood bank, to begin the process as well as ending the process. Communication of worsening patient condition or crisis must be prompt and clear. Communication methods include notification of the surgical team of the escalating events and closed-loop communication among team members. Closed-loop communication can be described as a transmission model in which verbal feedback is of great importance to ensure that the team members correctly understand the message.[11] The communication strategy commonly involves 3 steps, with an implied step of repeating back information for confirmation of accuracy (**Fig. 1**):

1. The sender conveys the message
2. The receiver acknowledges receipt and repeats back/reads back the information using numeric or phonetic tools
3. The sender acknowledges the accuracy of the repeat-back by confirming.

Another facet of MTP is maintaining accuracy and organization of documentation in the blood bank and clinical area. The following methods are used to assist with organization in the blood bank and patient care area:

1. Prepare packs in advance of the need to prevent delays in transfusion support
2. Use of numbered packs
3. Color-code blood product labels based on pack number
4. Provide transfusion tracking forms ("pack sheets") with the blood
5. Keep track of the number of packs dispensed with the blood bank tracking form.

Clinical staff also must maintain accurate and organized documentation of the fluid volume, blood transfusion administration, and patient assessments. Because transfusion is an integral part of the process, simulation of the processes was imperative to ensure safe administration of blood products. "Pack sheets" (Appendix 1) were incorporated with the coolers of blood products for staff to keep count of the blood products administered and to ensure the intended ratio of blood products was maintained. In addition, staff had the opportunity to manage transfusion support resources, such

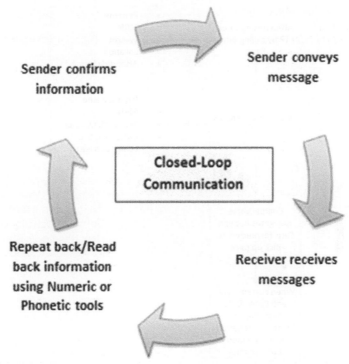

Fig. 1. Closed-loop communication.

as the level 1 rapid infuser, the Enflow blood warmer, and the POCT devices used to monitor laboratory values as the MTP progresses.

The people resources involved in the MTP, must also be secured and organized. The role of the floor charge nurse is for resource management and delegation of workflow. The simulation team also used the clinical administration supervisor to assist staff in finding people resources throughout the hospital who could both assist in caring for patient needs as well as staff who could go to blood bank to retrieve blood product packs (**Fig. 2**).

RESULTS

During the prebrief, the facilitator reviewed the expectations, objectives, capabilities of the patient simulator, and the equipment necessary for the event. At this stage, the staff was informed that they should treat the simulated patient or "manikin" as a live postoperative patient with spinal fusion who was hemorrhaging, requiring the MTP. The intent of the extensive prebrief was to provide basis of a psychologically safe learning environment.[12] The goal was to ensure that staff knew that they were free to make mistakes and to push the boundaries of their professional knowledge and skills. During the debriefing, the facilitator again established a safe environment by first giving positive reinforcement regarding the confidentiality surrounding their performance to the simulation participants.

After creating the psychologically safe learning and discussion space, an adaptation of the Gather-Analyze-Summarize (G.A.S.) debriefing tool was used immediately after the simulation event. This allowed time for feedback of what went well, and what could

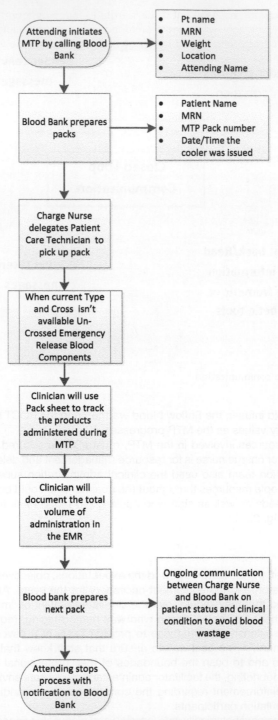

Fig. 2. MTP algorithm. EMR, electronic medical record; MRN, medical record number; Pt, patient.

be improved, to include assessment of deliberate practice, outcome measurement, simulation fidelity, skill acquisition and maintenance, and team training.[13] During the initial phase, the participants voiced that they had little experience with high-fidelity manikins and simulation scenarios that incorporated high degrees of realism with the integration of unfamiliar processes. For example, they expressed the feeling of uncertainty with the realism of carrying out the interventions of actually infusing blood products and fluids into the simulated patient. This feeling of uncertainty existed despite the comprehensive prebriefing. The facilitation team was diligent in enacting a psychologically safe environment, which allowed learners the opportunity to express their concerns and discomfort without fear of reprisal. This led to identification of barriers, including concerns about availability and location of equipment, limited staffing, limited experience with acute procedures, and discomfort with existing processes.

In the next phase of debriefing, curriculum integration was introduced. High-risk complications of surgery, including hemorrhage in patients with spinal fusion, were reviewed. Staff had the opportunity to ask questions, and education was provided as well as discussion surrounding available resources for future use. This was also a time to identify infrequently used clinical skills identified during this simulation, including the push-pull method of rapid blood administration, techniques to warm blood, and monitoring laboratory tests for unintended consequence of MTP, among others. Operational skills acquisition and reinforcement included documentation, ordering, and crisis resource management in a critical event. Although the census of spinal fusion surgeries is low in this small hospital and hemorrhage is a low-volume high-risk complication to the spinal fusion surgery, we are able to translate the process of MTP to other diagnosis and acute events. This allowed for transfer of practice and reinforcement of skill acquisition.[5]

Team dynamics and cohesiveness were identified as the largest contributing factor of success, and greatest risk of adverse event to the patient, by the learners and supported by the facilitation team. One of the largest barriers, and greatest lesson learned, was the concept and application of critical crisis resource management. In this small PICU, staffing is limited to 4 to 5 nurses, including a charge nurse, a patient care technician, advanced practice provider, and an attending during the day. Learners were able to conceptualize the volume of team members needed to successfully complete MTP and what each role entailed. The importance of a strong formal leader was also identified as a key role in the process. Situational awareness was discussed at length, as the team continued to develop a comfort for a fluid process. The organization, tempo, and flow of the room and care provided to the patient were debriefed as the participants shared what worked and what did not. A lack of close-looped communication prohibited the team to fully understand the roles that each person was fulfilling and the status of the patient after each intervention. Utilization of unfamiliar equipment posed a barrier, and Universal Protocol was a factor when participants did not follow it and were removed from the scenario and sent to "Occupational Health" per the health system's protocol. Finally, documentation was discussed at length, as the team struggled with identifying a designated recorder who was proficient in comprehensive documentation in a critical incident. Subject matter experts discussed the importance of flow and content of input and output in MTP and how the lack of proper documentation could lead to complications for the patient. Methods, legal responsibility, and efficiency also were topics in this conversation.

At the conclusion of the simulation, several adjustments were made to the blood bank process so as to effectively meet the caregiver and patient needs in a timely manner. Because the patient and surgery date are known, the blood bank temporarily increases the par stock levels of red blood cells to make sure staff has sufficient stock on hand to support the potential massive transfusion on the surgery day or in the 3 days after surgery. The blood product inventory level check form was revised to include a section for massive transfusion patients to ensure the stock was ordered from the supplier. The blood bank also found that they could improve the speed at which the first pack could be delivered by preparing it in advance for the patient. Because the patient is known, the staff are able to crossmatch red blood cells and have ABORh-compatible thawed plasma and platelets available for immediate release should an event occur. As soon as the first pack is released, the procedure is to prepare the next pack so that the staff can stay 1 pack ahead and do not delay the patient transfusion support.

SUMMARY

With the impending arrival of patients with spinal fusion, it became apparent that the PICU staff would need to be proficient with the activation and implementation of the MTP. Through the lens of the objectives, the teams successfully recognized the indications that warranted the triggering of the MTP. However, as expected, they also displayed discomfort working through the unfamiliar process of the MTP, which included using specific equipment and crisis resource management. The collaboration between all affected departments presented a unique opportunity to identify and modify processes that will better support the MTP. The blood bank made process revisions to increase the speed of getting necessary blood products to the patient, with all processes having since been implemented.

In conclusion, this simulation provided the PICU and blood bank staff the opportunity to have the actual setting in which the complex process of MTP could be practiced in a safe environment. This not only yielded latent system issues, but it also created a safe forum that allowed the learners to improve skills and provide feedback resulting in process changes that may improve patient outcomes in any area of the hospital that triggers the MTP. Each department and discipline in this simulation has had an opportunity to evaluate their role within this process. By using the simulation as a diagnostic tool to test operational readiness and closing knowledge gaps, they increased their confidence and skill for caring for their future pediatric patients with spinal fusion. In total, 3 simulations were conducted. One was videotaped for reference and future educational purposes. Although initially a post-test was not given to participants, a test has since been created for future simulation events with MTP to help assess educational decay and the appropriate time frame for refresher training (Appendix 2).

REFERENCES

1. Karam O, Tucci M. Massive transfusion in children. Transfus Med Rev 2016;30: 213–6.
2. Porteous J. Massive transfusion protocol: standardizing care to improve patient outcomes. ORNAC J 2015;33(2):13–30.
3. Institute of Medicine (US) Committee on Quality of Health Care in America. Errors in health care: a leading cause of death and injury. In: Kohn LT, Corrigan JM, Donaldson MS, editors. To err is human: building a safer health system. Washington, DC: National Academies Press; 2000. p. 26–43.
4. Lopreiato JO, Downing DK, Gammon W, et al, editors. Healthcare simulation dictionary. Rockville (MD): Agency for Healthcare Research and Quality; 2016. AHRQ Publication No. 16(17)-0043.
5. Cheng A, Duff J, Grant E, et al. Simulation in paediatrics: an educational revolution. Paediatr Child Health 2007;12(6):465–8.

6. Rudolph JR, Simon R, Rivard P, et al. Debriefing with good judgment: combining rigorous feedback with genuine inquiry. Anesthesiol Clin 2007;25(2):361–76.

7. Hunt EA, Shilkofski NA, Stavroudis TA, et al. Simulation: translation to improved team performance. Anesthesiol Clin 2007;25(2):301–19.

8. Hunt EA, Nelson KL, Shilkofski NA. Simulation in medicine: addressing patient safety and improving the interface between healthcare providers and medical technology. Biomed Instrum Technol 2006;40(5):399–404.

9. Children's Health System of Texas. Massive Transfusion Protocol. 2016. Published internal document.

10. Armstrong P. Bloom's Taxonomy. Nashville (TN): Center for Education, Vanderbilt University. Available at: https://cft.vanderbilt.edu/guides-sub-pages/blooms-taxonomy/2016. Accessed November 21, 2016.

11. Härgestam M, Lindkvist M, Brulin C, et al. Communication in interdisciplinary teams: exploring closed-loop communication during in situ trauma team training. BMJ Open 2013;3(10):e003525.

12. Rudolph JW, Raemer DB, Simon R. Establishing a safe container for learning in simulation: the role of the presimulation briefing. Simul Healthc 2014;9(6):339–43.

13. Phrampus PE, O'Donnell JM. Debriefing using a structured and supported approach. In: Levin AI, editor. The comprehensive textbook of healthcare simulation. New York: Springer Science+Business Media; 2013. p. 73–4.

APPENDIX 1: MTP PACK SHEET

MTP Pack Sheet

CAREGIVER MASSIVE TRANSFUSION PROTOCOL WORKSHEET

NOT PART OF THE MEDICAL RECORD.
All transfused units must be recorded on the "Record of Blood Administration" form.

Patient Name:	
Medical Record #:	
Patient Weight:	
Date/Time:	

MTP Patient Guideline

☐ Patient weight <10kg	1:1 ratio of PRBCs, thawed plasma, and platelets
☐ Patient weight 10 – 40kg	2 PRBCs, 1 thawed plasma, 1 platelet Consider 5 cryoprecipitate every other pack starting with pack 2
☐ Patient weight >40kg	5 PRBCs, 3 thawed plasma, 1 platelet Consider 10 cryoprecipitate every other pack starting with pack 2

Pack #	Transfused PRBCs Unit Numbers	Time	Transfused Thawed Plasma Unit Numbers	Time	Transfused Platelets Unit Numbers	Time	Transfused Cryo Unit Numbers	Time
1	_____	___	_____	___	_____	___	_____	___
2	_____	___	_____	___	_____	___	_____	___
3	_____	___	_____	___	_____	___	_____	___
4	_____	___						
5	_____	___						

Date and Time Next Pack Initiated	Date:	Time:
Administrative Supervisor Notified	Date:	Time:
Nurse Completing Documentation (Print Name)		

APPENDIX 2: MTP POST-TEST.

1. How do you initiate the MTP with the Blood Bank?
   a. Dial 0 and tell the operator you need blood
   b. Dial the emergency 3333 and ask them to transfer you to Blood Bank
   c. Dial 34867 and give them pertinent patient information
   d. Have the provider put in an MTP order in EPIC

2. What information do you need to give Blood Bank when you initiate MTP?
   a. Pt name, room number, way find #, diagnosis
   b. MRN, CSN, Pt name, DOB
   c. Pt name, diagnosis, weight, and MD
   d. Pt name, MRN, Weight, Location, Attending MD

3. In the ICU how does the cooler of blood products arrive to the unit?
   a. The blood bank tubes each if the different blood products
   b. A clinical tech or designee goes to the blood bank to pick it up
   c. A blood bank employee will deliver the cooler to the unit
   d. The charge nurse yells at that one nurse that you know is not busy to go get it

4. Blood Bank packs a cooler containing the appropriate blood products based on weight and labels the cooler with which of the following:
   a. Pt name
   b. MRN
   c. MTP pack number
   d. Date/time cooler was issued
   e. All of the above

5. In the simulation scenario the patient weighed 38kg, based on this information we can expect that the blood cooler will contain which of the following:
   a. 1 unit PRBC, 1 unit Thawed Plasma, 1-unit Apheresis Platelets
   b. 2 units PRBC's, 1 unit Thawed Plasma, 1-unit Apheresis Platelets, 5 units Cryoprecipitate (with 2nd cooler)
   c. 5 units PRBC's, 3 units Plasma, 1 platelets, 10 units Cryoprecipitate

6. It is acceptable to warm Platelets and Cryoprecipitate
   a. True
   b. False

7. It is acceptable to warm PRBC's and Platelets
   a. True
   b. False

8. While it is recommended that the products provided in the MTP pack be administered per protocol, the attending medical staff member may opt to request additional products not originally provided in the pack and/ or to not transfuse components for the MTP pack.
   a. True
   b. False

9. Which of the following is NOT true regarding use of the Level 1 Rapid Infuser?
   a. Must be used on 20g IV or larger
   b. Patient must be > 25 kg
   c. A RN is designated to run the level 1 with no other duties
   d. It is recommended to use trifurcate tubing in case you need additional med lines

10. When is it recommended that you change out the tubing on the Level 1 Rapid Infuser?
    a. When you can't figure out why the machine is alarming
    b. Every 24 hours
    c. After the 3rd blood product infused via the Level 1
    d. Sometime before the end of your shift

11. After the first MTP pack has been delivered/picked up, the Blood Bank prepares the next pack and will continue to do so until they are directed by the Attending Medical Staff member or designee to stop
   a. True
   b. False

12. Achieving normothermia is a critical component of adequate resuscitation, in the MTP sim scenario, in what order did the team utilize warming methods for their patient?
   a. Bear Hugger, Level 1, Enflow
   b. Bear Hugger, Enflow, Level 1
   c. The team failed to adequately

13. Cartridges for the Enflow fluid warmer and Tubing for the Level 1 Infuser are kept:
   a. In the ER Omnicell
   b. You have to get them directly from distribution
   c. In ICU Omnicell
   d. Both a and c

14. In the simulation scenario, when the second blood cooler arrives, what can the team expect to be different in this pack?
   a. Nothing, it is exactly the same as the first pack
   b. It contains only PRBC's
   c. In addition to the products in the first pack, it will include 3 units of Cryoprecipitate
   d. It contains only Platelets

15. In a patient such as the one in our scenario, what would be the fastest way to obtain H/H?
   a. I-Stat Cartridge G-4
   b. Send a specimen to lab with STAT as priority
   c. Utilize the Hemocue POCT located on the unit
   d. Take a guess based on how pale the patient is

16. You can NOT initiate MTP on a patient without a valid type and cross
   a. True
   b. False

17. You need an EPIC MD order to initiate MTP
   a. True
   b. False

18. When the blood cooler arrives what component should be given first?
   a. Platelets
   b. PRBC's
   c. FFP
   d. The provider determines most appropriate product based on pt. clinical status

19. How are the blood packs/coolers labeled when they arrive to the unit?
   a. Each cooler will be labeled with the color dot and pack #
   b. Everything inside the cooler will be labeled with the same color dot
   c. Both A and B
   d. None of the above, there is no way to keep track of the packs

20. I have watched the MTP simulation video and read MTP protocol 2.09
   a. True
   b. False

Abbreviations: DOB, date of birth; EMR, electronic medical record; ER, emergency room; H/H, hemoglobin/hematocrit; ICU, intensive care unit; IV, intravenous; MD, Medical Doctor, physician; MRN, medical record number; POCT, point of care testing; Pt, patient; PRBC, packed red blood cells; RN, registered nurse.

Moving?

Make sure your subscription moves with you!

To notify us of your new address, find your **Clinics Account Number** (located on your mailing label above your name), and contact customer service at:

Email: journalscustomerservice-usa@elsevier.com

800-654-2452 (subscribers in the U.S. & Canada)
314-447-8871 (subscribers outside of the U.S. & Canada)

Fax number: 314-447-8029

Elsevier Health Sciences Division
Subscription Customer Service
3251 Riverport Lane
Maryland Heights, MO 63043

*To ensure uninterrupted delivery of your subscription, please notify us at least 4 weeks in advance of move.

Printed and bound by CPI Group (UK) Ltd, Croydon, CR0 4YY

07/10/2024

01040506-0010